VIBRATIONAL NUTRITION

"*Vibrational Nutrition* is a joy to explore. You will learn to develop your sixth sense about food with Candice Covington as your mystical guide to the edible plant kingdom! In my practice of medicine and Ayurveda, I teach clients that food is more than calories and nutrients to be tallied—it is energy and information—and this book explores the depth of that understanding on an energetic and vibrational level that can help us to understand our own food cravings and aversions and how foods can affect our mood, behaviors, and our spirit. What a delicious delight!"

VALENCIA PORTER, M.D., M.P.H.,
AUTHOR OF *RESILIENT HEALTH*

"Candice is a true alchemist of nature! Her ability is like no other to translate the language of the plant world, through wisdom that surely spans lifetimes, with an eloquence in her words that is smooth like velvet. This book and the lifetimes of wisdom within its pages are the spiritual blueprint for understanding food at its most expansive and energetic level. Candice provides readers an entirely unique and, in many cases, previously unexplored viewpoint on 'who' are the specific foods that we consume."

AMANDA REE, LEAD EDUCATOR, EVENT HOST,
AND LEADERSHIP TEAM MEMBER AT THE CHOPRA CENTER
FOR WELLBEING AND FOUNDER OF SAMA DOG

VIBRATIONAL
NUTRITION

Understanding the
Energetic Signature of Foods

CANDICE COVINGTON

Healing Arts Press
Rochester, Vermont

Healing Arts Press
One Park Street
Rochester, Vermont 05767
www.HealingArtsPress.com

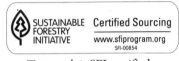

Text stock is SFI certified

Healing Arts Press is a division of Inner Traditions International

Note to the reader: *This book is intended as an informational guide. The remedies,
approaches, and techniques described herein are meant to supplement, and not to be a
substitute for, professional medical care or treatment. They should not be used to treat a
serious ailment without prior consultation with a qualified health care professional.*

Cataloging-in-Publication Data for this title is available from the Library of Congress

ISBN 978-1-62055-917-8 (print)
ISBN 978-1-62055-918-5 (ebook)

Printed and bound in the United States by Lake Book Manufacturing, Inc.
The text stock is SFI certified. The Sustainable Forestry Initiative® program promotes
sustainable forest management.

10 9 8 7 6 5 4 3 2 1

Text design and layout by Virginia Scott Bowman
This book was typeset in Garamond Premier Pro, Legacy Sans, and Gill Sans with
Fruitger and Ostrich Sans used as display typefaces

To send correspondence to the author of this book, mail a first-class letter to the
author c/o Inner Traditions • Bear & Company, One Park Street, Rochester, VT
05767, and we will forward the communication, or contact the author directly at
www.divinearchetypes.org.

In loving appreciation, I dedicate this book to my grandmothers,
Edna and Edra, to my mother, Sandra, and to all the women in my
family who came before them, and to Mother Nature,
for the wealth of wisdom they have shared with me
in my cellular memory, in my personal experiences,
and around the table. I thank you.

I would also like to thank the Cook family, especially
Curtis and Charlotte; my parents, Sandra and Harold; Maureen;
my wonderful editors, Jamaica Burns Griffin and Margaret Jones;
my darling duck and goose children; and my beautiful garden
for being endlessly supportive.

Contents

Preface

My love of the earth and her healing essences, in all forms, comes in part from my maternal line. My great-great-great-great-grandmother Griffith was a folk-wisdom herbalist, healer, and midwife in a frontier town in central Utah, where she practiced and took care of the women in her community.

My grandmother Edra, whose name means "powerful," was indeed a powerful woman of the woods and the earth. Some of my earliest memories of her are of going mushrooming. She would pack up my two sisters and me and take us to untamed places in the Rocky Mountains, hunting for wild mushrooms. I still remember her, with her Filson hat firmly pinned in place, wearing a peachy-orange lipstick, looking quite the lady in jodhpurs and white button-down shirt. I recall her loading us grade-school kids into a hand-over-hand pull tram that she somehow managed to find in the deep overgrowth of mountain trees. She would pull us across the river far below, and I remember looking down into that yawning canyon as the water raced its way through sharp rocks. Even at that tender age I admired her for being so sure-footed as she navigated us through such intimidating terrain. She always knew exactly where the tastiest treats could be found, like morel mushrooms, all wrinkly and wise. She would cook pounds of them in a simple sauté of butter, garlic, and fresh sage from her garden.

It is so fascinating to look at the energetic qualities of the foods that stand out at certain times of our lives, the foods that help shape who we are. As you work with this system I suggest you keep a journal and write down life events and the foods that stood out at those specific times. This will allow you to travel back in time and see how you have co-created with nature.

Morel Mushroom: A miraculous gift of spring and of the moist forest, morel invites you into the deep mystery where secrets and wisdom lie, opening you to the energy of prophecy, magic, and portents of your life to come. It enables a more comprehensive view of reality and the ability to enter into a visionary state to gain a more comprehensive view of reality.

My grandmother could have used any herb, but she consistently picked sage.

Sage: This herb is a master cleanser and purifier that can nullify all discordant energy. This doesn't mean it's permanently removed—you still have to do your personal work to shift the cause of the disharmony—but sage can offer refuge and hold space for you while you do so.

Garlic: Garlic brings the energy of affirming the divine light that dwells in your core, and using this inexhaustible source to warm your soul. In this light you are protected from negative energy and malevolent forces and granted the ability to protect others. Garlic also offers the gift of respecting the freedom of those you love, teaching by example and holding space for others to find their way without pushing them along before they're ready.

Reading the energy of my grandmother's recipe for sautéed morels, I see that it instilled in me the ability to abide in deep mystery and learn how to listen and interact with my surroundings in a subtle way, while holding the energetic space for me to learn at my own pace and be completely protected while I did so.

As a child I didn't realize what a delicacy morels were because when they were in season we enjoyed them in such great abundance. Grandmother so loved nature she would bring it inside—she grew white button mushrooms in the dark, mysterious depths of her closet. If I close my eyes I can return to the memory of me climbing into her closet, crawling on hands and knees toward a frosted window at the back of her wardrobe. There, under hanging pants, skirts, and blouses, where her shoes should have been, I would plant myself in the dark, loamy-scented air, allowing my eyes to adjust in the dim light until I could see the otherworldly bumps of white mushrooms pushing their way up into the world. It was an enticing mix of Chanel No. 5, earth, decay, and growth. I didn't realize it then, but my grandmother was paying homage to the balance of nature in all of her forms. She taught me without words to travel inward, to the darkness, to find the growth that comes from decay, and to not be afraid of it but instead to rejoice in the mysteries of life and nature.

She also took us south, to the high desert of Utah, to gather pine nuts, which energetically promote the energy of profound self-love. She would have us spread large white sheets under the trees, after which she would beat the limbs of the trees with a broomstick to get the pine cones to fall. I still remember the scent of the pine resin on my hands, which would linger for days. We explored the rugged landscape carved from wind and weather, the dry, hot air filled with the scent of sagebrush, cedar, and juniper. She taught me to take in the beauty of the land around us and listen to the silent stories it told. We would take the pine nuts back to her home to roast on large baking sheets in the oven, the scent filling the house with the bounty of Mother Earth's gifts. It was not until much later that I realized that she not only offered me my first wildcrafting experiences, she also revealed to me, through touch, taste, scent, and sight, the sunny, bright spirit aspects of nature and the dark, moist, soulful aspects, without ever saying a word about how each half made a perfect whole.

IN THE BEGINNING: DREAMING INTO REALITY

My invitation from the Divine to write this book came in a most unexpected way, in a series of dreams knocking on my awareness to open the door of my conscious mind wide enough to understand what nature wanted me to do.

This is the first dream that awakened me to this project. I have done very little editing and have tried to keep the details just as they were presented to me, as I feel it's important to follow the narrative of what the Divine was communicating to me.

I am in a large underground room painted a cream color, with no furniture (it is light and I can see). The only object in the room is a smoky-green velvet curtain that covers an entire wall. A wind comes through the space, and I can see the curtain move, and then I can feel the wind moving through me. I don't like that—it scares me and I try to think of a mantra that would expel it. For a while I just stand there searching my memories. I pull a mantra to mind and know it's incorrect, so I try another one and another one until I realize that I don't know one that will work.

I then ball my fists up and yell into the room "I command you to be gone!" Immediately, a man, Charles, whom I know in real life (he's an engineer, which I equate with the left brain, being precise and practical), appears. I tell him what's going on and that I need him to help me. He picks up a dark-haired woman with long, flowing hair and starts spinning her in circles (a circle is one of the yantras—sacred geometry—for the air element). I watch and wonder why he's doing that instead of using sage/ smudge, as she is not going to get rid of anything. In the next part of the dream (after I come to awareness, which is often referred to as witness consciousness *in dreaming), I am watching Charles spin the woman around and I start to think as I watch, and the first thing that comes to mind is how it "feels" when fresh thoughts come in, and why it's so hard for me to get authentically new information or insights, because when they come I try with all my might to reject them. It also occurs to me that the smoky-green curtain (a teaching symbol) represents air (smoky green is the color I associate with that element, and I could see the curtain rippling) in my normal thought process, so I recognize what's being communicated to me.*

I am a longtime student of alchemical traditions, and this how I understand the function of the element air:

- Carries and facilitates positive change, relates to the intuitive body
- Promotes curiosity, learning, and flexibility on all levels
- Allows the mind to achieve new insights and fresh perspectives
- Associated with abstract understanding and dreaming; the element of active dreamers, the visualization of what could be
- Promotes freedom from attachments (dogmatic, emotional, mental, and so forth)
- Supports shifting and directing consciousness, and swiftness in all forms
- Bridges the mundane and the Divine

I came to understand that the eerie wind that unnerved me is what inspiration actually feels like. Charles, the rational mind aspect of me, is trying to integrate the flow of information that's being fed to me instead of rejecting it, despite loud protests from another part of me.

This was a numinous dream: my muse was trying to communicate something entirely new to me, but I was unwittingly blocking her, and she wanted in!

My next dream made clear what she wanted. Again, I didn't edit the dream, as I feel it's important to listen to what's being conveyed instead of having it match a desired narrative.

I enter an abandoned fast-food restaurant, and all the tables are covered with refuse—old trays with crumpled-up wrappers, half-eaten food, etc. I start to clean the place up, and then suddenly I'm sitting in a lecture hall, and a male teacher whom I admire is lecturing on the nutritional value of fish and what types we should eat. I raise my hand and ask, "Shouldn't we determine the type of fish we need by first understanding what our personal matter is made up of?" He says, "Yes," and invites me to move down to the front row. I do, and then he invites me to sit on his lap, which I do. I sit chest-to-chest with him and wrap my legs around his waist (the exact same position as a traditional Tibetan Buddhist yab-yum). He then takes my shirt off and starts to rub a rough-textured plant paste on my breasts, and then suckles my nipples. I'm worried that my breasts aren't good enough and say as much. Looking down at them I see they are withered and small, but then they became full, ripe, and beautiful. I enjoy the feeling and really want to continue, but I know he's married and I'm married (in waking life this is not true, it's symbolic), so I feel we should stop. I say, "We're going to get in trouble, we'd better stop this." Then he moves us to an out-of-the-way corner and lays me on the floor and unbuttons my shirt again and applies the same paste and starts to suckle my breasts again. This time I feel a more intense pleasure. I really like it and want him to continue, but I'm distracted because I'm worried about being caught by his wife. So I ask him to stop, and he does.

Sure enough, I didn't dream in this same vein for months, until my psyche had time to process this information. What I came to understand was that I was being asked to create from a feminine intuitive place something concerning the role of food at a subtle level, and subconsciously I felt I would "get in trouble" on some level from critics for not having verifiable information that I could point to as a precedent. I was also having difficulty having new thoughts because I was "wed" to old thought systems that I had spent my whole life studying (still equally true). The fascinating part of human incarnation is that so many things are equally true at the same time, and it was time for me to learn in a new way, to get my succor (i.e., "suckle") directly from Mother Nature's breasts, instead of someone else laying down the information in my mind. So I am truly excited to share what is included in this book, where it is my intention to offer some additional tools from nature that can support us in the spirit of love.

Deepening Our Relationship with Food

Nowadays most everyone is familiar with the unique health benefits of fruits, vegetables, protein, herbs, and spices and their specific effects on the human organism. For example, it's now widely known that turmeric is a powerful anti-inflammatory, that lemon supports optimal liver function, that carrots significantly improve eye health, and so on. I have always been mindful of how certain foods stimulate my body, but as I have deepened my relationship with and understanding of food, a fascinating new layer has started to unfurl.

I am a longtime student of Ayurveda as well as flower essences, plants, and esoteric aromatherapy, and so I've developed a good foundation for understanding the subtle body. Through this work I was led to understand how my food cravings and aversions revealed a fascinating story of me at the most subtle level—what I refer to as my *deep self.* I discovered that I was leveraging the world around me through the food choices I was making to construct specific states of being, both positive and negative. This is a radical concept, so allow me to elaborate.

Early in life I had a strong distaste for yellow crookneck squash. Reason told me it was because I didn't like the texture or taste. However, as I came to understand the *energy signature* of food, I realized there was a more significant explanation. I don't like structure or routine, and because that is exactly the energy that yellow crookneck squash brings, I avoided this plant altogether! As I've matured and adopted a more conventional routine, I now actually crave the way it supports my productivity and organization, and so I regularly incorporate it in my diet.

> Quantum physics asserts that everything has a vibrational nature. Of course, this applies to the food we consume as nutrition. And each type of food, just like each person's handwritten signature, reveals unique energetic properties that point to its nature and "personality." This distinct vibrational nature of the different foods we eat is its *energy signature*.

I can also reflect on a certain period in my life when I couldn't eat enough mussels. At the time when my craving was at its peak, I was struggling with clearing a deeply rooted past-life karma that was manifesting as an emotional state—in this case, anger. I couldn't understand why this anger was coming up because I couldn't point to anything in my life that would cause me to feel this way. It was quite an unconscious craving for this shellfish at the time, but I now understand that the food signature of mussels acts to alleviate anger. My deep self knew the remedy I needed to help me in my time of difficulty.

In this book we will explore the energy signatures of more than 400 of the common foods we eat and how they help form the vibrational structures that influence us on the mental, emotional, and spiritual levels. You'll gain a deep understanding of why you crave certain foods and dislike others and thus be able to consciously craft a diet to support you in any endeavor. As you become familiar with each food profile, you'll notice that each plant, animal, legume, herb, spice, and grain has a slightly different "voice." Some are more lyrical. Some are serious. Others are mystical. Each food has a unique way of expressing its energetic gift. Some voices will naturally resonate with you, and others you may dislike. It's possible that only certain aspects of each energy signature will apply to you at any given time. Remember, this is only one piece of the puzzle, as you are constantly shifting and evolving. You may crave different foods purely for their physical health benefits, and others you may choose to omit due to their unfavorable effects on your physical body or belief system.

Nature holds real magic, and not just a sleight-of-hand attempt to fool the mind. As you become more deeply aware of this magic, you'll be able to consciously work with and use the constructs of nature to bring about specific states of being. My own relationship with the magic of nature began with a singular prayer in my heart. Ever since I can remember, in every ritual, group activity (no matter the tradition), and prayer I have asked for one thing: that the plant kingdom teach me directly, without the middleman. I have studied many different schools of thought from many great minds and traditions concerning plants and their applications, but I wanted more.

When it finally happened, it was unexpected and I was broadsided. I was sitting on my bed reading *Jane Eyre* when all of a sudden, before my waking eyes, luminous yellow twin buttercup fairies about the size of my thumb appeared and laid down these words in my mind: *"We are here to heal you."* They then entered my body through my chest area and I saw many interconnecting light lines in different hues against an indescribable background. My awareness was enfolded in this light, what I'm guessing is my energy body, and then *true bliss* filled my body. I had read about the sensation of bliss, but until this moment I had never felt it personally. I can testify, it is beyond words. These miniature beings then took me from consciousness while they did their work, and just as suddenly they brought me back. The transition was more immediate than waking from sleep. They then appeared before me and said that they would help me see. As they entered my forehead, images and information rushed in. I felt deeply afraid and overwhelmed, and I told them so. They stopped and left immediately. I have wished every day since that I had been braver and allowed myself to see what would have happened.

Years went by and my fairy friends never returned for a waking visit, though I began having numinous teaching dreams that guided every aspect of my learning and creating life. I could not wait to fall asleep each night. I was so fascinated with the change in my dreams that I started seeing a Jungian analyst who specializes in dream analysis to help me drill down into what I should do with this newfound gift. After some soul searching, I found that I wanted to collate the information I was receiving and share it with the world. Not long after, I had a dream about my grandmother that inspired me to start writing in earnest. I was alone in my paternal grandmother's kitchen, standing in front of her stove with a pot of pumpkin soup simmering away. Suddenly, the stove gave way and opened like a doorway, with stone steps that led down, down, down into welcoming darkness. I knew from my dream that pumpkin was a way I could connect to my deceased grandmother and start on my path of working with ancestral knowledge.

As I got to know the beings of the plant kingdom—through my dreaming life as well as my waking life as an aromatherapist, gardener, and cook—our relationship bloomed into a rich friendship that feels like family. One of the most dynamic ways of connecting to the energetic beings of nature is to actually use the plant kingdom to entrain your matter and energy to a frequency that will make it easy for them to communicate with you. For instance, as we will learn in this book, violet flower can help you connect with the fairy realm, purple plum radish supports clarity and vividness in dreams, the grain teff helps nature beings speak directly to you through symbols, and borage flower enhances your ability to have visions.

These days, when I receive information about a plant or a food, it usually bubbles up like an epiphany. Each presents differently, but I receive a strong knowing coupled with great excitement and bodily sensations. I think my fairy visitors created this way of experiencing the world for me. I am grateful to them for doing so, and grateful to be able to share this world with you.

Each chapter in this book concludes with an exercise such as the following one, intended to help you build your knowledge about the vibrational nature of food and how to apply that knowledge. The self-assessment exercise here is an excellent starting point for accessing the energetic bodies of the food you eat. One of the goals of this book is to develop our "sixth sense" so that we can learn how to relate to our fellow beings (yes, vegetables are beings too!) that we take in as food as a way of understanding our interconnectedness with Mother Nature. As you progress through each chapter, you'll see how you can work with food to affect your mood, your behavior, and your spirit. I recommend taking this quiz every so often to check in and see which foods currently most support you, or why certain foods were meaningful to you at some point in the past. Then, read the energy signatures for each of these items described in chapter 1, and compare your first impressions to the descriptions found there, which are based on my own explorations and those of my students. In chapter 2 I describe my discovery of my own "food familiar," and in so doing I hope to show you how to find yours. In chapter 3 we'll be looking at how food shows up in our dreams and how to cultivate an awareness of the messages that different foods give us in the dream state that we can apply to our daily lives. In chapter 4 you'll learn more about how the colors of foods relate to the function of the different chakras, and how to strengthen certain energies or tone them down as needed. Chapter 5 demonstrates how to create your own "food narratives," and in chapter 6 you'll find a collection of recipes organized by energetic states.

So dive in, and in this way you'll gain insight into the vibrational nature of your current diet and make any changes or adjustments to fine-tune your energetic body, removing negative energy patterns and consciously crafting a positive state for body, mind, and soul through the nutrition you take in.

SELF-ASSESSMENT
Tuning In to the Energy of Food

Before you read about the energetic signatures of foods listed in the next chapter, take time to tune in intuitively to the energy of each to get an unbiased reading. Ground and clear your mind and set your intention to "read" the vibration of each food. Avoid recalling past experiences that are flavor-based, and instead feel into the energetic signature. Please try to keep an open mind if something seems odd, or if honestly you would never eat the food (acknowledge that but keep with the energetic sensation). Allow food to be an oracle alerting you to some aspect of yourself that would benefit from your attention.

As the writer Tom Robbins says, "There are only two mantras, yum and yuck." This is obviously not strictly true, but in the context of exploring the concept I am putting forward here it's the perfect set of mantras to help answer the question at hand. When doing this exercise it's important not to get caught up in your mind, but just allow your intuition to flow, going with your first impression, or your gut instinct, so to speak. Select only items you get a strong charge from, either feeling drawn to or put off by. Place a plus (+) sign next to foods you feel drawn to and a minus (–) sign next to foods that are not appealing. Note that frequently a strong dislike of a food signifies an imbalance of some sort, something that you subconsciously resist changing in your life. On the other hand, foods you are drawn to eating often illuminate either traits that are very "you" or qualities your higher self wants you to cultivate.

Vegetables

Artichoke

Arugula/Rocket

Asparagus

Bean, Green

Bean, Yellow Wax

Beet/Beetroot

Beet Greens

Broccoli

Broccoli Rabe/Rapini

Brussels Sprouts

Cabbage

Carrot

Carrot Greens

Cauliflower

Celery

Celery Root/Celeriac

Corn

   Country Gentleman (Sweet)

   Glass Gem (Popcorn)

   Golden Bantam (Sweet)

   Picasso (Sweet)

   Ruby Queen (Sweet)

   Shaman's Blue (Popcorn)

   Wild Violet (Sweet)

Cucumber

Eggplant

Endive

Fennel Bulb

Frisée

Garlic

Garlic Scapes

Heart of Palm

Jerusalem Artichoke/Sunchoke

Jicama

Kale

Kohlrabi

Leek

Lettuce

   Butter

   Iceberg

   Romaine

   Spotted Trout

Lotus Root

Mizuna/Spider Mustard

Mushroom

   Chanterelle

   Cremini

   Enoki

   Hedgehog

   Hen of the Woods/

     Maitake

   Lion's Mane

   Lobster

   Morel

   Oyster

   Porcini/King Bolete

   Portobello/Portabella

   Royal Trumpet

   Shiitake

   Truffle

   White Button

Okra

Onion

Parsnip

Pea

   English

   Snap

   Snow

Pepper

   Anaheim

   Ancho

   Banana

   Bell

   Cayenne

   Chipotle

   Ghost

   Habanero

   Hatch Chile

   Jalapeño

   Padrón

   Peppadew

   Pepperoncino

   Poblano

   Scotch Bonnet

   Serrano

   Tabasco

   Thai/Bird's Eye Chili

Potato

   Fingerling

   Purple/Blue

   Red

   Russet

   White

   Yukon Gold

Pumpkin

Radicchio

Radish

   Black Spanish

   Daikon

Fruits

Avocado

Banana

Berry

   Blackberry

   Blackberry, Himalayan

   Black Currant

   Blueberry

   Cloudberry

   Cranberry

   Elderberry

   Goji Berry

   Gooseberry

   Huckleberry

   Marionberry

   Raspberry

   Strawberry

Caper

Cherry

Citrus

   Bergamot

   Blood Orange

   Citron/Buddha's Hand

   Common Orange

   Grapefruit

   Kumquat

   Lemon

   Lime

   Mandarin Orange

   Tangerine

Coconut

Date

Dragon Fruit/Pitaya

Fig

Grape

Guava

Kiwi Fruit

Mango

Melon

   Cantaloupe

   Honeydew

   Watermelon

Nectarine

Olive

Papaya

Passion Fruit

Peach

Pear

Persimmon, Fuyu

Pineapple

Plantain

Plum

Pluot

Pomegranate

Pomelo/Pummelo

Prickly Pear

Quince

Star Fruit

Tamarind

Wildcrafted Plants and Edible Flowers

   Borage Flower

   Caper Flower

   Carnation Flower Petals

   Cedar Leaf Tips and Branches

   Chamomile Flower

Dandelion

Elderflower

Fiddlehead Fern

Johnny-Jump-Up and
 Pansy

Lilac Flower

Marigold Flower

Nasturtium Flower

Nasturtium Leaf

Nettle, Purple Dead

Nettle, Stinging

Purslane

Queen Anne's Lace

Red Clover

Rose Hip

Rose Petal

Saint-John's-Wort

Violet

Finishing Salts

Fleur de Sel

Himalayan Pink Salt

Kilauea Onyx Sea Salt

Molokai Red Sea Salt

Herbs and Spices

Allspice

Asafoetida

Basil

Bay Leaf

Black Pepper

Caraway Seed

Cardamom

Celery Seed

Chicory Root

Chive

Cilantro Leaf

Cinnamon

Clove

Coriander

Cubeb

Cumin

Dill

Fennel Seed

Fenugreek

Filé Powder

Galangal

Ginger Root

Grains of Paradise

Horseradish

Juniper Berry

Kaffir Lime Leaf

Lemongrass

Mace

Marjoram

Mint

Mustard Seed

Nutmeg

Oregano

Paprika

Parsley

Peppermint

Pink Pepper Seed

Rosemary

Saffron

Sage

Star Anise

Summer Savory

Tarragon

Thyme

Turmeric

Vanilla

Grains

Barley, Pearl

Buckwheat

Bulgur Wheat

Farro

Millet

Oatmeal

Quinoa

Rice

   Arborio

   Basmati

   Brown

   Forbidden

   Jasmine

   White

   Wild

Rye

Teff

Wheat, Bread/Hard Red

   Winter

Wheat, Durum

Legumes and Beans

Anasazi Bean

Black Bean

Black-Eyed Pea

Butter Bean

Cannellini Bean

Chickpea/Garbanzo Bean

Edamame

Fava Bean

Flageolet Bean

Gigante Bean

Kidney Bean

Lentil

Lima Bean

Lupini Bean

Navy Bean

Orca Bean/Calypso Bean/

   Yin-Yang Bean

Peanut

Pinto Bean

Red Bean

Nuts and Seeds

Almond

Brazil Nut

Cashew Nut

Chestnut

Chia Seed

Cocoa "Bean"

Flaxseed

Hazelnut

Hemp Seed

Macadamia Nut

Pecan Nut

Pine Nut

Pistachio Nut

Poppy Seed

Pumpkin Seed

Sesame Seed

Sunflower Seed

Dairy

Camel Milk

Cow Milk

Goat Milk

Sheep Milk

Water Buffalo Milk

Yak Milk

Eggs

Black-Headed Gull Egg

Chicken Egg

Duck Egg

Emu Egg

Goose Egg

Guinea Hen Egg

Ostrich Egg

Quail Egg

Fish

Alaska Pollock

Anchovy

Arctic Char

Barramundi

Catfish

Cod

Halibut

Lingcod

Mahi-Mahi

Monkfish

Perch

Rainbow Runner

Rainbow Trout

Red Snapper

Rockfish

Salmon

Sand Dab

Sardine

Sea Bass

Shark

Sheepshead

Sole

Squid

Swordfish

Tuna

Shellfish

Abalone

Clam

Butter

Geoduck

Razor

Venus

Cockle

Conch

Crab

Crayfish/Crawdad

Langostino

Lobster

Lobster, Spiny/Rock

Mussel

Oyster

Scallop

Sea Urchin

Shrimp

Fowl

Chicken

Duck

Goose

Grouse

Ostrich

Pheasant

Quail

Turkey

Other Proteins

Beef

Boar/Wild Pig

Elk

Goat

Lamb

Pork/Domesticated Pig

Rabbit

Seitan/Wheat Gluten

Tempeh

Tofu/Bean Curd

Venison

Beverages

Coffee

Tea

    Black

    Green

    Oolong

    Pu-erh

    White

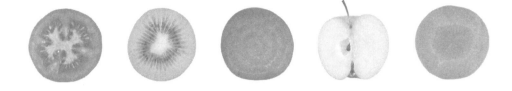

1

The Frequency of Food

Energetic Signatures of More Than 400 Foods

If more of us valued food and cheer and song above hoarded gold, it would be a merrier world.

J. R. R. TOLKIEN

The natural world, with its vast and wondrous array of forms and energies, offers a treasure trove of vibrational tools that we can use as antidotes for negative energy patterns and to support the cultivation of positive qualities. As noted earlier, the vibration of each plant and animal can be understood as an energy pattern with a specific and unique structure or signature. When these energetic signatures resonate with our natural vibrational patterns, we can use them to fine-tune our energetic bodies.

As Jungian analyst Edward C. Whitmont states, "Every pattern of adaptation, outer and inner, is maintained in essentially the same unaltered form and anxiously defended against change until an equally strong or stronger impulse is able to displace it."* The energetic signature of each plant and animal offers the architecture of a stable foundation onto which we can consciously craft our inner world and thereby transform our outer reality. Because we are vibrational beings in a con-

---

*Whitmont, *The Symbolic Quest*, 246.

stant state of flux, a significant key to our well-being and growth is the reinforcement of our desired energetic patterns.

Food is such an effective medium for holding matter at specific vibratory rates, and the foods included in this book have energetic signatures that I have gotten to know intimately and have relied on over the years. This is such a simple and effective way to support your whole being. Food nourishes every aspect of well-being, from being one of the most dynamic ways to sustain your physical health to creating and maintaining even the subtlest aspects of the self—the mind, emotions, soul, and spirit.

THE ETHICS OF EATING RESPONSIBLY

The Golden Rule, "Do unto others as you would have them do unto you," refers to treating others the way you want to be treated. This applies to our food, those living beings—vegetable, animal, and mineral—that provide us with nourishment and sustain our physical, emotional, mental, and spiritual energy. And if you truly accept that we are individual manifestations of the same whole, embodying one another in a state of interconnectedness, then it makes sense that you wouldn't want to harm any other living being any more than you would consider harming yourself.

> Plants offer the gift of transmuting light into life through photosynthesis—liquid emerald. In essence, this is the Emerald Tablet of the ancient alchemists, which opens us to the esoteric concept "As above, so below," and teaches us how to learn from this eternal wellspring.

Cultures from around the world have eaten everything you can think of: from peoples in the Far North, who mostly had a meat diet due to harsh weather; to peoples who are vegetarian or vegan due to belief; to peoples who believe hunting is sacred; to peoples who developed in fertile areas that were prosperous and peaceful, who focused on food as art and ate a little bit of everything. In modern times there have been endless scientific studies telling us the right way to eat. I think diet is incredibly personal, and there is not any one correct way to approach diet outside of this important dictum: *Be kind, and do it with reverence.*

Let's start esoterically and work our way down to the physical. It's important to understand that *food is memory.* Mother Earth has been refining herself from the beginning of time; every species of plant and animal has contributed to her evolution. Each carrot, deer, marigold, etc., possesses a cosmic memory, has a unique story to tell, and reflects the light of the universe, which in turn helps us remember our own origins and evolution. Humankind as a microcosm contains within itself all of the elemental kingdoms—mineral, plant, and animal.

Plant Power

Plants are a divine boon and greatly influence us on a subtle level, kneading and forming our energetic bodies by linking our physical self with nature's divine intelligence. Plants continually configure the feeling self, which can be understood as the phenomenal aspects of our emotional, spiritual, and mental lives. The more you ingest a specific plant, the more its energetic signature becomes your energetic signature. Once it is understood how plants inform so much of our behaviors, the question becomes, how do you want to treat this plant creator of you that you will consume? I would say mindfully engage with plants with the greatest respect and reverence and do what you can to create an ideal living situation for them. The grace of the plant kingdom will aid you regardless, but if you want to forge a relationship, put forward actions that will cultivate connection.

The Sanskrit word for plant is *osadhi,* which loosely translated means "a burning transformation that occurs in the receptacle of the mind."

There is now a wonderful trend toward supporting small local farms, as evidenced by the farm-to-table movement and the proliferation of farmers' markets. These are not merely places to shop for food; they are considered outings that rival going to a museum. Many people keep their own gardens, showing great creativity in growing food in small outdoor spaces or in containers. This tells me that people want to connect with their food personally; they understand that the happier the plant, the more dynamic its prana, or chi, will be. At farmers' markets you'll often find heirloom varieties, which is especially exciting because food is memory, and this allows you to tap into historical options, thus ensuring that biodiversity continues and we do not lose these unique plant beings and their knowledge.

Today we find more and more organic options that reduce our risk of exposure to harmful pesticides. Dr. Valencia Porter, a leader in environmental and preventive medicine, states:

> Organophosphate pesticides (OPs) were originally developed as neurological poisons for chemical warfare in World War I and act as a poison to the nervous systems of insects, plants, and humans. High levels of OPs are associated with increased ADHD, decreased IQ, and dementia. A different class, called *organochlorine pesticides,* poison insulin-receptor sites, worsen metabolic syndrome and diabetes, and have other effects on hormonal and immune systems. The herbicide atrazine, found in 94 percent of our water supply, has been linked to birth defects, infertility, and cancer. Combinations of these chemicals with other toxic agents such as arsenic and aluminum can have synergistic effects, making matters worse. The good news is that blood levels of these toxins can decrease quickly after switching to organic foods.*

If pesticides affect us this harshly on a physical level, not to mention their subtle effects on us, just try feeling into the experience of a plant that is continually poisoned from birth to harvest. This is not a nourished or

---

*Porter, *Resilient Health,* 51.

nourishing space. It's no way to treat our fellow beings of the plant realm.

One thing I hear about a lot is that certain foods have a "high vibration" and are ranked as so-called superfoods because of their supposed extra potency. However, I think it's important not to put one fruit or vegetable above another; they all serve a vital role. I would encourage you to look at the plant kingdom in its completeness as an energetic medicine chest. A few rules of thumb do apply, however, for keeping your produce vibrant and radiant: the fresher the better, as more of its vital energy is still intact; grown with love from a source you know; organic if at all possible; and once at home, handle with love and attention. Finally, take time to give thanks and show your respect when you store your produce, prepare it, and cook it.

If you cannot swing it to buy local, organic, lovingly raised produce, please do not stress or judge yourself. If you live in an area with fewer options or if financially it's not possible to obtain these premium foods, do the best you can with what you have at your disposal, and always give thanks and show respect.

Animal Husbandry

The same principles that apply to vegetables apply to the animal products we consume. The quality of life for farm animals and the land on which they are raised are paramount when it comes to the energetic value of the food they provide us with. On a purely physical level, when antibiotics and added hormones are introduced into your body via poor treatment of animals and land, as in factory-farm situations, it's more than likely that your meat was exposed to bacteria and viruses and inhumane living conditions. And it's well known that factory farms pollute the environment and poison drinking water, and as more of these animals must be fed, this means more industrial farming practices that introduce toxic chemicals into the land and waterways. On the other hand, free-range, pastured animals raised on natural forage supplemented with healthy food have a higher nutritional value, taste better, and offer numerous well-documented health benefits.

Let's talk about ethics. The members of the animal kingdom wear their hearts on their sleeves, so to speak, and they are a direct reflection of we humans in that they feel things physically and emotionally. They have complex inner lives, family structures, and unique languages and personalities. How can we not shower them with love and care? Ask yourself, "What do I need to thrive?" Of course we need plenty of space; balanced, nutritious food; a comfortable shelter; a family unit that is happy and where we feel safe and loved; and the chance to enjoy life. If this is so for we humans, then shouldn't we provide the same to those animals we consume as food? A unique role we have as human beings on this interconnected planet is to be stewards of the many animals who do not have free-will choice like we humans do.

There is spiritual wisdom to be found in "all our relations," including different animals, who can be our teachers and guides and help us understand our place in the cosmos. Many belief systems state that not only can we learn from animals through observation, prayer, and study, but they also teach us behaviors and lessons on a subtle level when we take them into our bodies as physical nourishment. There is a strong ethical consideration and responsibility when it comes to the energetics of the animal products we consume. Beyond the physical and environmental concerns, beef from a factory farm, for instance, does not provide the same energy as pastured beef humanely raised and slaughtered.

Jamie Sams, a member of the Wolf Clan Teaching Lodge, reminds us how paramount it is to give other beings their space, be it protecting wild habitats or promoting proper animal husbandry: "Nature teaches us how to know ourselves in the purest way possible. If we listen and watch, every lesson of human living is given by the animals, the changes in the Wind, Father Sky, Mother Earth, and All Our Relations. Each aspect of your world has its space in which to create. If that space is respected by others, growth continues in harmony."*

It is important to remember that you take into yourself not only all

---

*Sams, *Sacred Path Cards,* 319.

the cosmic memories but also cellular memories from the meat, dairy, and eggs you consume. It is vital that you gather all from an ethical and humane source, as their memories and emotions become your memories and emotions.

I live in rural Oregon, where small farms, hobby farms, and homesteading are common. Here it's easy to source meat, eggs, and dairy from people who have devoted their lives to mindful and loving animal husbandry and stewardship of the land. Even if you live in a city, increasingly there are options for choosing ethically and sustainably sourced animal products, whether at the local farmers' market or at a natural foods store, and nowadays, in response to a growing movement recognizing the health benefits of eating humanely raised animals, some large supermarket chains are offering pasture-raised products. So wherever you live, try your best to source your meat, eggs, and dairy from a source you trust.

Energetically, animals as the food we eat teach us within the active principle. Their gift is to refine the mind and bring forth the act of discrimination, which allows us to perceive and make judgments. Within this lens we can weigh what is true and false, good and bad, real or unreal, valuable or worthless. This vibration allows us to observe our circumstances and separate the wheat from the chaff, leaving us with the truth of a situation.

Processed Foods and Other No-No's

Processed foods have a bad rap, but in reality any time we cook, bake, or prepare food, we're processing it. There is the prewashed and bagged lettuce or spinach (preferably organic) that we use for convenience's sake, or precooked whole grains, Greek yogurt, nut butters, organic stock, tofu, frozen vegetables, and unsalted canned beans—all acceptable from a vibrational standpoint. In contrast to these benign forms of processing is the other end of the spectrum—foods that have been heavily altered with chemical preservatives and damaging, questionable, rancid ingredients and added colorings; snacks that come in packages with a long list of unpronounceable additives; pre-made microwavable meals; and frozen pizza. These foods, as you probably have guessed, are energetically "dead" and to be avoided.

Refined sugar is another taboo in vibrational nutrition. It is extracted from foods like corn and sugar beets (which are usually genetically modified crops) and sugar cane. The chemically produced sugar that results from the extraction process, including the worst, high-fructose corn syrup, is added to foods and beverages such as crackers, packaged cereals, flavored yogurt, tomato sauce, and salad dressings. Low-fat foods are the worst offenders, as manufacturers consistently use refined sugar to add flavor. Most processed junk foods add calories and unhealthy forms of sugar and have no nutritional value, in contrast to natural forms of sugar such as fruit and unsweetened milk, which have vitamins and minerals, fiber, and protein. As well, a diet of junk food is not only dead in terms of nutritional value, it is also a leading cause of cancer, heart disease, diabetes, and other ailments of our modern, "civilized" society.

Following Oscar Wilde's dictum "Everything in moderation, including moderation," I do use certain processed foods in moderation in my cooking, including canned tomato paste, anchovy paste, canned unsalted beans, jarred artichoke hearts, olives, tofu, soy sauce, and so on. These items obviously do not offer as much chi or nutritional value as their fresh counterparts, but they still carry the energetic blueprint from the foods they hail from. For example, you want to explore the energy of pinto beans, you could use either dried or canned unsalted beans to access that frequency.

The final word on processed foods is this: as embodied beings, pleasure has a role in our lives. Cooking for the sake of the taste experience or making a recipe exactly the way your mother made it offers certain pleasures that makes our lives fun. Needless to say, if any of these foods cause harm or contribute to an imbalance or disease, you should eliminate them from your diet.*

---

*Remember, I'm writing from an energetic point of view, so if you're interested specifically in how food impacts your physical health, especially if you have food allergies or specific health problems, I recommend *Resilient Health* by Valencia Porter and *Perfect Health* by Deepak Chopra.

◆◆◆

It is such a rewarding and life-affirming practice to get to know the foods we eat a little bit better! What follows is just a glimpse into how each behaves based on my own experience and interactions. Plants and the other foods we eat are incredibly complex and have many expressions of self. The *Rig-Veda* (10.97.2) famously celebrates this, stating, "Mothers [plants], you have a hundred forms and a thousand growths. You who have a hundred ways of working, make this man whole for me." Our foods offer a multifaceted range of gifts. I encourage you to take the following descriptions as a jumping-off point to deepen your own relationship with and knowledge of each food.

VEGETABLES

Vegetables, in the broadest sense, include any kind of plant life. The term usually refers to the edible portions—roots, stems, and leaves—of certain herbaceous plants generally prepared in savory rather than sweet dishes. Energetically, vegetables offer stability, foundation, and structure to our lives.

Artichoke

This variety of a species of thistle supports mental functioning to delve into higher dimensions, those beyond what is usually available. For many people this extends to the fifth dimension, where we can open to receiving communications from our guides and spirit helpers. Artichoke helps us assimilate messages of a channeled nature, particularly those that are otherwise difficult to understand.

Arugula/Rocket

This tart, peppery, leafy member of the Brassicaceae family enhances the ability to bring order to chaos and to have light, simplicity, and harmony at your center, from which all activity unfolds. It brings focus, will, and concentration derived from your higher self.

Asparagus

This spearlike plant, a springtime treat, expands your subtle perception so you can see more clearly the energetic information coming from others, allowing more harmonious interactions and supporting healthy relationships. What is hidden comes into plain view. It is also supportive in dispelling depression, abandonment issues, abuse, and fear and dynamic for honing discernment and setting boundaries.

> Asparagus releases debris from the aura—fears and prejudices—setting you free from the grip of powerful presences like strong parental figures, cultural conditioning, power struggles in relationships, and so on.

Bean, Green

With pods that are either green or purple, this plant fosters creativity and the fulfillment of desires and teaches perseverance in the face of obstacles so you can learn your lessons with as much ease as possible. It softens your struggles and helps you see their value in your life, allowing you to take a breath of fresh air and face your fears, especially the vulnerable aspects that are intensely personal.

Bean, Yellow Wax

Wax beans teach natural magic that allows you to tap into your deepest gifts and dance with them in ecstasy until those gifts blossom into their fullest expression.

Beet/Beetroot

The beet is the ancient ancestor of the autumn moon, bearded, buried, all but fossilized; the dark green sails of the grounded moon-boat stitched with veins of primordial plasma; the kite string that once connected the moon to the Earth now a muddy whisker drilling desperately for rubies.

TOM ROBBINS, *JITTERBUG PERFUME*

This intense vegetable opens the door to your inner realms, including past-life recall, and supports the conscious mind in exploring many aspects of the self previously unknown, restoring and integrating these aspects for use in daily life.

Beet Greens

The leaves of the beet plant can help you keep with your long-term goals with faith, perseverance, and endurance.

Broccoli

This member of the Brassicaceae family offers the gift of achieving balance, helping you to be responsible and respond to the challenges you face. Broccoli also helps you "get it right" and clear up loose ends that nag at you internally, like taking care of unkept promises and unfulfilled duties, including those that matter to others.

> Broccoli helps you choose your tasks with freedom and joy, so your to-do list comes from a place of service. This is accomplished by allowing you to tap into the fullness of your mind and your robust energy.

Broccoli Rabe/Rapini

The leaves, buds, and stem of this plant, which somewhat resembles its cousin, broccoli, release rigid or negative thought patterns that keep you stuck and often result in emotional and physical disorders such as a stiff neck, back or knee problems, etc. It's good for those who tend to be critical and judgmental. It restores joy and spontaneity, allowing you to become gentler and more open to the ideas and wishes of others.

Brussels Sprouts

These miniature cabbages that grow on a single stem promote the gift of finding and expressing valuable details and expressing a genius for the unusual, the ability to discover valuable information and find innovative applications for this knowledge.

Cabbage

Both purple and green varieties help heal the sensation of loss of success or abundance and feelings that because you didn't succeed in the past you cannot succeed in the future. They support the need for individuality and a life-path direction informed by the soul.

Carrot

Coming in a variety of colors (orange, yellow, red, white, purple, black), the carrot offers support if you tend to overanalyze, worry excessively, and get caught up in "what ifs" to the point that it becomes a personal detriment. It's important to be judicious when you weigh what's in front of you; carrot offers the gift of being able to see what's an imaginary fear and what's a healthy concern.

Carrot Greens

The Bugs Bunny–like foliage of the carrot offers the gift of breaking down crystallized patterns. Are you in a rut? Do you have habits or attitudes that no longer serve you? Carrot greens can help dissolve those walls to allow new life in, and since this can be unnerving, the greens also offer the inner support needed to make your transformation not so startling.

Cauliflower

Cauliflower clears the energy of the family tree (on both sides), both prebirth and in utero, creating a neutral energy that can be consciously worked with by the parents to set intentions and blessings for their new baby. It also creates space for the incarnating child to remember past-life lessons and incarnate with awareness and will. Eaten by an adult, it clarifies cellular memories stored in the body.

Celery

Celery, currently enjoying a wellness boom for its physical benefits, is also bursting with vital energetic values. It nourishes your prana, and in doing so it restores depleted energy, strength, and balance, especially when you're under pressure. Celery allows your body to be nourished by your soul's commitment to life. This plant also helps you understand what changes need to be made to cultivate greater well-being, along with the will to follow through on your inner knowing.

Celery Root/Celeriac

Scrub celery root with a stiff brush under cold running water and trim the root end. Peel away the thick skin as deeply as needed to remove any brown furrows.

To remain steadfast and able to maintain your viewpoint against opposition, take celery root, the bulbous knob of a variety of celery grown for its edible stem and shoots. Celery root allows you to accept experiences labeled "crazy" or that are unexplainable so you can integrate them into your life, while expanding your ability to examine these experiences from a higher perspective and see the meaning they give to your life, knowing you need no outside verification, as you already have inner knowing.

Corn (General)

Corn, which comes in a multitude of varieties and colors, brings fertility and supports alignment with the earth's energies, opening you to the cornucopia that life offers and providing an earthy groundedness. A sacred plant of Native Americans, it ushers in abundance on all levels, especially the joy and pleasure associated with the feminine. Corn supports increased creativity and birthing the projects that result, and it is useful for fostering friendships and associations based on mutual support and growth by promoting the synergy needed to achieve goals larger than your own. See specific corn varieties beginning on page 38.

Corn as we know it today would not exist if it were not for the peoples of Mesoamerica who domesticated it from a grass called teosinte approximately ten thousand years ago. A human innovation, corn does not exist naturally in the wild and can only survive if planted and protected by humans. Conversely, the budding human race would not have been able to develop without the stability corn provided. Humans and corn have a truly symbiotic relationship, and there are numerous legends and creation stories about how corn came into being and how it served and protected the people, bringing abundance.

Cucumber

"Cool as a cucumber" describes the energetic essence and vibrational action of this plant, which offers broad-spectrum relief for easing difficult emotional states. It can be understood as nature's own Rescue Remedy,* as it refreshes and renews the physical body after exhaustion, illness, and shock, while deeply supporting you in reengaging with life.

I went on holiday and put self-watering bulbs in my potted plants on my front porch. The weather was much warmer than predicted, and I came home to some very sad plants. I knew they needed more than plain water. I ran my hand over various fruits and vegetables, asking the question "What will help my plants recover?" and feeling for the strongest vibration. They picked cucumber and said to apply it for a week, and they would return to their vital, strong health. So I cut slices of cucumber and let them soak for at least 20 minutes in the vessel I use to water my plants with.

Eggplant

> *Kindness is more important than wisdom, and the recognition of this is the beginning of wisdom.*
>
> THEODORE ISAAC RUBIN

---

*Rescue Remedy, probably the most well known of the Bach flower remedies, is an all-purpose remedy for emergencies, crises, and stress. It's a blend of flower essences: impatiens, star of Bethlehem, cherry plum, rock rose, and clematis.

Eggplant is an invitation to remember that once you have reached the pinnacle of prowess, success, and security, it is wise to share your good fortune with others. This can take many forms, so how this expresses itself is up to you and your soul. Generosity will always come back to you a thousandfold if it is gifted with selfless goodwill.

Endive

A member of the chicory family, which includes radicchio, escarole, frisée, and curly endive, this leafy plant helps you keep your integrity and self-respect and supports you in staying faithful to your own inner knowing.

Fennel Bulb

This flowering member of the carrot family assists those weary of life and lacking creative imagination and energy; it facilitates attunement to higher realms and reawakens the creative impulse.

Frisée

Frizzy frisée is helpful for those who hide their true feelings out of a sense of shame; it promotes emotional honesty through the release of shame.

Garlic

Garlic brings the energy of affirming the divine light that dwells in your core, and using this inexhaustible source to warm your soul. In this light you are protected from negative energy and malevolent forces and granted the ability to protect others. Garlic also offers the gift of respecting the freedom of those you love, teaching by example and holding space for others to find their way without pushing them along before they're ready.

Garlic Scapes

The tender stem and flower of the hardneck garlic plant helps heal myopic states, when you can't see the forest for the trees.

Heart of Palm

The heart or core of certain palm trees holds the matrix and pattern of lightness and freedom, interlacing plates of energy within your being.

Jerusalem Artichoke/Sunchoke

This species of sunflower creates a sense of relating to and understanding what is occurring on Mother Earth politically, geologically, and emotionally, and it brings a greater awareness of Earth as Gaia, a living being, as it nourishes the desire to live in harmony with all of creation.

Jicama

This potato-like root vegetable brings a burst of new energy, alerting you to new possibilities that are open to you now and inviting you to start afresh, make new plans, hatch new ideas, and open to the rising inspiration that is available right now.

Kale

Kale, a leaf cabbage, offers instruction in remembrance by passing on skills, wisdom, and ancestral knowledge and teaching you how to use this information in new ways. This is a result of being a receptive and porous student, gleaning family history and your own cellular remembering, and, finally, offering the information and understanding you have collected to others. An aspect of this is being able to clearly articulate your thoughts, being a receptive listener, and engaging in fruitful debates of ideas and exploring concepts with others. These aspects together make for a very good teacher and student indeed.

It's no wonder that kale is the sweetheart of the yoga, meditation, and ancient philosophy set—on a subtle level this plant firmly supports these processes.

Kohlrabi

Also known as German turnip, this rather odd-looking plant, which must be peeled before eating, heals fear of punishment or criticism if you depart from the dogmatic beliefs of family or community and alleviates apprehension or avoidance of threshold experiences due to fear-based beliefs.

Leek

This member of the onion family helps you understand symbols and the complex nature and layers of information they contain. It assists you in interpreting the rich symbolism that makes up your life, including dream imagery, and helps you identify the projections around you so you can understand the quality of human togetherness at any particular time and place.

> Leek helps you determine where you're at in your evolution.

Lettuce (General)

A refreshing annual plant of the daisy family, *Lactuca sativa* has edible leaves that are a usual ingredient of salads. Energetically, lettuce bridges the mundane and the divine to foster love, forgiveness, and compassion. Many varieties have been developed with a range of form, texture, and color; most are cool-weather crops. See specific lettuce varieties beginning on page 39.

Lotus Root

The rhizome of the aquatic flowering lotus plant, lotus root is crunchy and delicate in flavor. Lotus holds the vibration of the entire path of enlightenment and is a powerful teacher and guide. This radiant plant first stimulates you at the unconscious level, bringing the desire to become self-actualized, and then supports this path as your budding consciousness learns the lessons offered from each chakra center. Of course, the ultimate goal of this plant is to usher you into a state of enlightenment. This is an excellent plant to reach for when you cannot quite name what has you stuck but you know that you need relief. Lotus supports your whole life journey and circumstances.

Mizuna/Spider Mustard

A leafy green belonging to the Brassicaceae or mustard family, mizuna has a peppery, piquant, and mildly bittersweet taste. It is supportive for the individual who has a hard time coping with the mundane and is locked into a routine or a job that could be perceived as drudgery. This vegetable can help you manage this energy until a shift can occur or help you make peace with the circumstances if it is a long-term situation that must be endured.

Mushroom (General)

The tissue of mushrooms—the fruiting bodies of certain species of higher fungi—consists of immense lengths of microscopic, threadlike hyphae and their aggregations, known as mycelium, which grow in soils or organic debris and in association with plant roots. We now know that these threads act as a kind of underground internet, linking the roots of different plants and allowing them to communicate. Energetically, mushrooms promote interspecies communication and act as a bridge linking us to multiple ways of knowing and enabling interaction with different realities. See specific mushroom varieties beginning on page 40.

Okra

Descriptively called "ladies' fingers," okra strengthens you so you're not pressured against your will or overly influenced by the desires of others who focus on you. It is an excellent plant to help heal dominant/submissive relationships.

Onion

Onion's many layers allow you to access the many layers of your being, letting you explore your vast energies. Do you want to work with a specific aspect of self? Clear a painful memory? Revisit a feeling? This vegetable is a gateway to any part of yourself, positive or negative, that you need to get at—all you need do is set your intention as to where you want to go and why.

Parsnip

This member of the parsley family helps foster a sense of independence and detachment without feelings of isolation.

Pea (General)

Snow, snap, and English peas are all climbing plants and members of the legume family, but there are subtle differences between the three. See pea varieties beginning on page 44.

Pepper (General)

Pepper (*Capsicum*) is a genus of more than thirty species of flowering plants in the nightshade family, Solanaceae. Many are extensively cultivated for their edible, often pungent fruits, which come in varied forms—from mild bell peppers that are used as a vegetable to hot peppers, such as habanero and tabasco, that are frequently used in hot sauces and relishes and pickled or ground into a fine powder for use as a spice. Energetically, peppers frequently instill passion, enthusiasm, and warmth. See specific pepper varieties beginning on page 44.

Potato (General)

> *What I say is that, if a man really likes potatoes, he must be a pretty decent sort of fellow.*
> A. A. MILNE, AUTHOR OF *WINNIE-THE-POOH*

The humble spud dramatically increases future sight, telepathy, clairvoyance, and the ability to use these gifts for healing, often resulting in practical solutions for everyday problems. This nightshade helps in assimilating and grounding you in the earth plane, allowing you to thrive. See specific potato varieties beginning on page 47.

Pumpkin

Whether or not you believe in morphic resonance, the ocean of archetypal memory from previous similar systems, pumpkin will connect you to the spiritual echo of past lives—not only to your ancestors, but to the universal wellspring of all who went before you, allowing you to see how closely we are linked to the past and how we are still driven by many of the same primal fears and needs faced by the first humans. The wisdom and teachings of our ancestors are freely available to us if you only ask.

Radicchio

This variety of the chicory plant is helpful for emotional stress or trauma, allowing a gentle relaxation so that the system can reintegrate before having to respond to the presenting situation. It allows you the ability to step back from things long enough to gather your inner resources and make space for proper decision-making.

Radish (General)

This hearty, easy-to-grow root vegetable replenishes the soul light held in the deepest structures of the body. Its gifts are generous: it supports recovery from drug and alcohol addiction with an infusion of hope and eases depression stored in the body as heaviness, listlessness, or flagging energy. This kind of energy frequently presents in the respiratory system and is often coupled with a sense of hopelessness or resignation; radish helps clear this. See specific radish varieties beginning on page 49.

Radish Greens

While the most commonly eaten portion of the radish is the taproot, the entire plant is edible and the tops can be used as a leaf vegetable.

Radish greens promote a strong self-contained individuality and celebrating your uniqueness rather than feeling isolated by it.

> The often-ignored radish greens are a powerhouse of nutrients, containing vitamin C, vitamin B6, magnesium, phosphorus, iron, calcium, vitamin A, potassium, and folic acid. They are believed to purify the blood, cleanse the liver, and flush out stored toxins. They have a wonderfully peppery bite that add panache to any dish and are equally delicious raw or cooked.

Rhubarb

With its reddish stalks and sour taste, rhubarb helps curb the need to be an exhibitionist, acting out inappropriate and intrusive behaviors in social settings to gain attention such as talking too much, being unaware of boundaries, and showing off. This plant supports shifting this kind of energy into feeling good enough as you are.

Rutabaga

A spheroid root vegetable that can grow to the size of your head, rutabaga helps you be calm, balanced, and centered within your higher self no matter what circumstances whirl around you, so you can hold your truth without force.

Scallion/Green Onion

Green onions bring you back in touch with your loved ones, promoting sensitivity. They help you to be in the here and now, patiently allowing time and space for closeness and the little joys of life when together.

> Scallions are helpful for busy parents, friends, and partners who find their distracted behavior is creating distance in relationships.

Spinach

One of the most nutritious foods on Earth, spinach supports you in nurturing yourself in a healthy way by fostering self-love, self-approval, and the ability for self-care. It's excellent for those who feel motherless, need mothering, or miss their mother's loving energy, as it opens you to the energy of the Great Mother.

Squash (General)

Squash in general are practical. They teach the ethic of "chop wood and carry water" and how to make it not a chore but a pleasure. They model earthly vitality, helping to integrate the more instinctual and bodily aspects of self. All forms of squash—and there are many, as these plants are prone to cross-pollination—arose in the Americas, primarily in the areas that are now Mexico and Central America. They are one of the Three Sisters crops, along with corn and beans; Native Americans found that when planted together these crops work in harmony to help one another thrive and survive. It is believed that they have been in cultivation for more than four thousand years. And while the body of the squash is edible, its seeds and blossoms are delicious also. See specific squash varieties beginning on page 50.

Squash Blossom

The bright yellow flower of the squash plant is excellent for prickly people who are always annoyed by something. This flower will soothe how you perceive the world and aids in not finding other people and certain circumstances so irritating. On the other hand, if you're in a situation where you have to communicate with a prickly person, squash blossom will take the edge off during exchanges, allowing you to stay calm and centered without feeling defensive.

Sweet Potato

A member of the morning glory family and not a nightshade, sweet potato clears the mind of all unnecessary thought, bringing stillness and silence, which allows adjustments to occur on a deep level. It is very supportive for meditation.

Swiss Chard

A relative of the beet, chard brings the awareness that you carry your home deep within you, where you may abide in peace and at-oneness. It is excellent for restoring this connection during periods of change when it's important to maintain your sense of self.

Tomato (General)

Tomato, first and foremost, teaches togetherness in many forms. Be it a loving family, a robust community, the dance of a relationship, a passion, or even courtship, this fruity vegetable is all about the heart. A part of this dynamic is its ability to help you be open to differences and new circumstances and joyfully embrace them. See specific tomato varieties beginning on page 51.

The age-old question—*Is a tomato a fruit or a vegetable?*—has an enjoyable answer: it is both. Tomatoes are fruits that are considered vegetables by nutritionists and chefs. British journalist Miles Kington amusingly said, "Knowledge is knowing that a tomato is a fruit. Wisdom is not putting it in a fruit salad." This debate made it all the way to the Supreme Court. In 1893, the high court was asked to rule on whether imported tomatoes should be taxed under the Tariff Act of 1883, which only applied to vegetables and not fruits. Justice Horace Gray summed up the ruling concisely: "Botanically speaking, tomatoes are the fruit of a vine, just as are cucumbers, squashes, beans, and peas." Although in the court's opinion, "In the common language of the people . . . all these are vegetables which are grown in kitchen gardens, and which, whether eaten cooked or raw, are, like potatoes, carrots, parsnips, turnips, beets, cauliflower, cabbage, celery, and lettuce, usually served at dinner in . . . the principal part of the repast, and not, like fruits generally, as dessert."* Pound that gavel, the verdict is in! In general, tomatoes are treated like a vegetable.

*Nix v. Hedden, 149 U.S. 304 (1893), available on Justia website, U.S. Supreme Court Center.

Turnip

Raw or cooked, turnips promote discrimination in all situations, helping you identify what is of use and what isn't.

Water Chestnut

A member of the sedge family, Cyperaceae, water chestnut is widely cultivated in Asia for its edible corms, which remain crisp even after being cooked. Water chestnut helps ease attitudes and perspectives that are too rigid and that create defensive behaviors, which prevent you from perceiving what is actually occurring.

Watercress

A cousin of kale and broccoli, watercress is an aquatic and semiaquatic green that's beneficial for those who are easily overstimulated by the ordinary events of day-to-day life. It facilitates flowing awareness and the ability to partake in life without being swept away by the sensorial aspects.

Yam, Jewel

I yam what I yam, and that's all what I yam.

POPEYE THE SAILORMAN

This starchy tuber facilitates the luminous expression of your unique creativity and inspiration, allowing your distinctive individuality to shine forth and enabling inspired acting and speaking in the world. Yam helps heal the inability to take social and creative risks and supports those experiencing midlife crisis by repatterning the soul forces and life expression.

❦ *Corn Varieties*

> While technically a fruit, corn is considered either a vegetable or a grain depending on when it is harvested. Fresh sweet corn, harvested when it is soft and has kernels full of liquid, is considered a vegetable. Corn that is harvested when fully mature and dry is considered a whole grain—this includes popcorn, though for simplicity I have included all of the corn varieties together.

Country Gentleman Sweet Corn

Unusual because its deep, narrow, white kernels are arranged irregularly, not in rows, this variety was developed around 1890 in the Connecticut River Valley. It helps heal all aspects of anxiety linked to perfectionism and softens worry about details. It helps you accept your present imperfect state.

Glass Gem Popcorn

With kernels beautiful enough to be stained glass—translucent, multicolored shades of blue, yellow, red, and everything in between—this particular variety was selected by Oklahoma farmer Carl Barnes, who began growing heirloom Native American varieties as a way to reconnect with his heritage. Energetically, this corn helps restore congruence between inner experiences and outer expressions.

Golden Bantam Sweet Corn

Developed in 1902, this yellow heirloom corn made yellow corn popular in the United States. Golden Bantam helps ground excessive, scattered energy to reestablish a natural and healthy flow that feeds activity without overstimulation. This allows you to feel in control of your life. It is very helpful if you can't sleep or relax because of frenetic energy.

Picasso Sweet Corn

Dazzling with its deep purple stalks and husks contrasting against white and yellow ears, Picasso sweet corn promotes an active and lively consciousness that is alert and flexible. This mobile state of mind allows you to celebrate the unique and unconventional. This corn can be very fun to eat in conjunction with creating or enjoying art, shopping at "junk" stores, looking for treasures, or watching offbeat films.

Ruby Queen Sweet Corn

A regal-looking corn with deep shades of vibrant red, this variety is as handsome as it is delicious, offering sweet, tender kernels. Ruby Queen supports your physical body, absorbing energy from the earth and bringing vibrant vitality. It can be used to address abundance issues and support financial stability.

Shaman's Blue Popcorn

Originating in the Andes Mountains of Peru, this variety has outstanding dark blue kernels, which almost look like gemstones. It helps focus spiritual energy for the development of the personality and supports integration after deeply transformational experiences.

Wild Violet Sweet Corn

A stunning bicolored corn with about 60 percent purple and 40 percent white kernels per cob, Wild Violet sweet corn helps activate your third eye and development of subtle perception. It brings penetrating insight and broadens your outlook, and it also helps you anchor this knowing into your body to help guide you. This corn is excellent to eat before journeying, prayer, or meditation.

❦ Lettuce Varieties

Butter Lettuce

Butter lettuce helps restore the milk of human kindness to your heart when you feel completely depleted and have nothing more to give (described often as feeling hollow inside) by connecting you to a source larger than yourself so that you can be refilled with a sense of compassion.

Iceberg Lettuce

Iceberg shifts the energy around unhealthy curiosity about the affairs of others and their personal information, which leads to gossiping, and helps bring the mind back to healthier, more balanced pursuits.

Romaine Lettuce

Romaine helps you drop the blame game and concentrate with greater sensitivity on the other person, allowing you to constructively focus on relationship building. One of the tools it offers is the ability to objectively self-analyze and apply this understanding.

Spotted Trout Lettuce

This lettuce variety supports replacing guilt with self-forgiveness, relieves related tensions, and fosters insight into behavior.

🍄 Mushroom Varieties

Chanterelle Mushroom

This aromatic, fleshy wild mushroom helps you shift the pattern of taking on too much responsibility (this looks different for everyone), pushing yourself too hard, and waking up early but feeling tired and not refreshed, leading to a dulling of the emotional body and the mind.

Cremini Mushroom

A cross between a white button and a portobello, cremini heals the energy of attacking the negative in yourself so that you can see and feel yourself in a gentler light, cultivating compassion for having those less-than-desirable traits and allowing kindness and softness to be a healing balm to relentless self-criticism.

Enoki Mushroom

This crunchy Japanese mushroom helps strengthen your emotional body so you don't become like the people who have let you down. It facilitates pulling yourself out of dependency/resentment cycles.

Hedgehog Mushroom

> *Hydnum umbilicatum* is commonly known as the hedgehog or sweet tooth mushroom due to having not gills but, instead, delightfully small, tooth-like projections that looks like hedgehog quills.

This sagely mushroom, easy to identify in the wild for its yellowish-orange cap and fruity scent, brings the strength and wisdom of the ages, reminding you to not act in haste and to understand the difference between knowledge and wisdom. Its gifts are generous: it gives you the patience to penetrate deeply into the heart of the matter and opens your spirit to consult those wiser than yourself, be they living elders, ancestors, or the wisdom recorded in books. This mushroom grants the strength and forbearance needed to slow down and consider motives and circumstances—your own and those of others—allowing you to take action only after thorough deliberation.

Hen of the Woods/Maitake Mushroom

This exquisite and often huge fungus found usually at the base of oak trees supports integrating and healing trauma by strengthening your willingness to look deeper and to face what has occurred in the past, coupling this with the ability to face life and understand the true reason for your reactivity. It helps clear feelings of overwhelm, confusion, resistance, and reactivity that often come when looking at old experiences. This can cause a disconnection in your energy field that makes you vulnerable to present-day experiences when confronted by a challenge to your sense of self. This mushroom supports you in rebuilding and strengthening your connection to your core and to your light body.

Lion's Mane Mushroom

Named for its large, shaggy appearance, this Asian specimen is notable for both culinary and medicinal uses. It encourages tenderness in those who fear to show that side of themselves lest they appear weak, a pattern that usually occurs as a result of societal indoctrination. Sadly, this can cause you to miss out on fully experiencing love and intimacy. Lion's mane can help right this wrong.

Lobster Mushroom

Not an actual mushroom but rather a parasitic fungus (with the color of a cooked lobster) that grows on certain species of mushrooms, this edible specimen grants the ability to observe your shadow side without feeling threatened so you can be emotionally self-nurturing, especially when outside support is not available.

Morel Mushroom

A miraculous gift of spring and of the moist forest, morel invites you into the deep mystery where secrets and wisdom lie, opening you to the energy of prophecy, magic, and portents of your life to come. It enables a more comprehensive view of reality and the ability to enter into a visionary state to gain a more comprehensive view of reality.

Oyster Mushroom

Coming with the fall season and growing wild on trees, this mushroom asks you to look inside and feel into what you believe you truly deserve in life. Do you really believe you have the right to be happy? Loved? Fulfilled? To follow your dreams? If so, the oyster mushroom helps you nourish those seeds further. If at a core level you do not harbor these kinds of feelings, you will be aided by this spirit ally in planting the seeds that will eventually allow you to actualize what your deep self requires to thrive.

Porcini/King Bolete Mushroom

This beloved and popular mushroom can help you explore the essence of true love that grows out of union with a beloved, whether it's your own inner self or another person. In this context, love means showing absolute concern coupled with the understanding of how to truly love yourself, allowing you to express empathy for another person.

Portobello/Portabella Mushroom

This mushroom helps you dwell in your center and not diminish the essential parts of yourself to make another person comfortable or happy. It supports you in defining your own needs while acknowledging others' needs.

Royal Trumpet Mushroom

Looking exactly like its name, this savory fungus instills consistency in achievement and energy output so you don't vacillate between doing too little and doing too much. It supports time management in all ways.

Shiitake Mushroom

A medicine and a culinary treat, shiitake promotes attunement to nature and helps you communicate with the plant and animal kingdoms. It can wake up entirely new forms of psychic energy with a sense of joy and wonder.

Truffle

The truffle supports being in the world but not of the world.

White Button Mushroom

The most prosaic of mushroom varieties can help you get centered in lightness and calmness despite rising pressures and tensions so that inner peace prevails. It supports you in seeing your options so you don't make life one long, hard choice.

❧ *Pea Varieties*

English Pea

With firm rounded pods, which are generally discarded, the round English pea brings you in touch with the softness of life, allowing deep empathy to flow from you. The hardened aspects of your emotional body become soft and supple again, and you are able to freely engage in the bright, uplifting side of your emotions.

Snap Pea

With an edible pod, crunchy texture, and very sweet flavor, snap pea helps clarify the difference between self-nurturing and self-indulgence.

Snow Pea

This tiny pea in an edible pod supports you in the full expression of emotions without being angered or provoked, bolstering a sense of detachment that allows harsh words to roll off your back so you can stop and think before reacting to hurt by creating more hurt.

❧ *Pepper Varieties*

Anaheim Pepper

This mild pepper can help you overcome resistance to change, being stuck in the past, and the energies of inertia, stagnation, and stubbornness, whether you are conscious of these patterns or not.

Ancho Pepper

A dried version of the poblano pepper, ancho helps you maintain your innocence, vulnerability, and sensitivity.

Banana Pepper

This mild pepper helps shift the energy of lust that blinds, and it dissipates delusional thinking, projections, and feelings of resentment and emotional insecurity.

Bell Pepper

One of the more fascinating aspects of the sweet bell pepper (in shades of green, red, yellow, and orange) is that it opens you to your wildness, to being untrammeled and not caring what others think of you. This sense of being completely natural allows you to grow the authentic aspects of yourself and follow goals that truly nurture you while lessening the fear of stepping into the unknown. It gives you the ability to be a cauldron unto yourself, a container in which to simmer everything you want to grow. Being such a sturdy vessel means gaining inner strength, resilience, and the ability to try, try, and try again until success is attained.

> One gift the bell pepper offers is letting you know when you should boldly and passionately follow your dreams, and when waiting in stillness for an opportunity to come to you is best. This can save a lot of headaches!

Cayenne Pepper

A hot pepper with many physical health benefits, cayenne is an invaluable aid in overcoming low vitality and exhaustion, physically and on an energetic level as well, when it cannot be replenished by rest alone.

Chipotle Pepper

A smoke-dried jalapeño, chipotle promotes alignment with the Earth from the ground up, especially through the feet and throughout the body.

Ghost Pepper

Considered one of the world's hottest peppers, this is the plant needed when your energy has been stunted to the point of not allowing yourself to dream, hope, or even plan a future that is anything but minimal and mundane—in short, for when you feel trapped in a cold, sterile, joyless life. Allow ghost pepper to warm and stir you, bringing new life in.

Habanero Pepper

A hot pepper that ripens to a vibrant orange or red, habanero can help you clarify your true feelings.

Hatch Chile Pepper

"Hatch" is a generic name for various types of chili peppers grown in the "pepper valley" of Hatch, New Mexico. It offers dynamic, effortless energy and lively activity coupled with inner ease.

Jalapeño Pepper

This hot specimen supports you in being centered in your own power and taking responsibility for your own life, moving from victim mentality to master of your destiny.

Padrón Pepper

This chili's energy is spicy and hot! It brings a full-blooded suggestiveness that encourages you to be physically passionate, expressive, and wild.

Peppadew Pepper

Trademarked under the Peppadew brand, this sweet cultivar enhances body-mind communication.

Pepperoncino Pepper

A sweet, mild Italian chili pepper, the pepperoncino enhances the ability to accept and absorb energy and be transformed by releasing outmoded patterns of behavior.

Poblano Pepper

This large, mild, heart-shaped pepper helps in the expression of emotions, especially if it's difficult for you to cry, reveal your pain, or ask for help.

Scotch Bonnet Pepper

Named for its resemblance to a Scotchman's traditional head apparel, this Jamaican pepper brings a strong sense of your inner conscience to guide you to be truthful and upright.

Serrano Pepper

This meaty little pepper promotes starlike, cosmic vision, which helps frame the events of ordinary life and put them in perspective.

Tabasco Pepper

This pungent pepper (after which the famous hot sauce is named) energizes and balances the first chakra and supports your ability to ground spiritual energy in the physical body. It can help you awaken to a higher, less personal, altruistic form of love.

Thai/Bird's Eye Chili

Hot and aromatic, this pepper balances psychic awareness with deep penetration and understanding of the transpersonal aspects of oneself.

❦ Potato Varieties

There are three basic potato types: *Starchy* potatoes are high in starch and low in moisture, and they have a floury texture with creamy white flesh. These are ideal for baking and not suitable for dishes that require boiling, roasting, or slicing. *Waxy* potatoes have less starch than starchy potatoes and contain more moisture and sugar. They hold their shape well after cooking and are great for boiling, roasting, and slicing. Since they hold their form, they are not ideal for mashing. *All-purpose* potatoes have a medium starch content that falls somewhere between starchy and waxy potatoes. As their name implies, they can be prepared with any cooking method and used in any dish. Although, if you have a specific recipe in mind, choose a potato type that best supports your dish. For instance, to make a baked potato, or jacket potato, you would choose a starchy potato to produce the fluffy interior that is desired.

Fingerling Potato

This all-purpose potato brings a deep awareness of your roots and supports connection to your family and soul group. It promotes the desire to create healthy communities by supporting farmers' markets, small local businesses, restaurants, musicians, and artisans.

Purple/Blue Potato

This all-purpose potato helps bring you into alignment with the wisdom of ancient civilizations. This may encourage you to find a teacher from the tradition you are drawn to, exploring your own cellar memories from your earliest roots. Or perhaps it will inspire travel to places that hold the earth energy you wish to explore.

Red Potato

This waxy potato helps heal the fear of commitment and supports you in putting down roots. It also assists you in keeping long-term friendships and helps ease the compulsion to bolt when things get difficult in romantic relationships.

Russet Potato

The starchy russet helps bring a deeper state of peace. It fosters an ability to set aside quarrelsome behavior and find a place inside your heart for greater understanding of others. It also provides motivation for humanity's continual endeavors to discover, to grow in humility, and to assist others.

White Potato

This all-purpose variety helps you become disciplined and keep a schedule. Allowing regularity in life helps you move forward and find your rhythm. It is a wonderful choice if you are prone to procrastination.

Yukon Gold Potato

This all-purpose potato helps you savor the richness of life. Bringing deep contentment to the here and now, it takes you deeper, allowing the fullness of the moment to envelop you.

❦ *Radish Varieties*

Black Spanish Radish

Cultivated since the sixteenth century, this radish has a deep, near-black skin and dramatically contrasting snowy white flesh. It is dynamic for clearing energies taken on from the environment, other people, and entities.

Daikon Radish

The daikon, whose name means "large root" in Japanese, ranges in size from six inches to three feet. It is beneficial for those who feel guilty because others are suffering and they are not.

French Breakfast Radish

This radish features vibrant coloring that graduates from a vivid fuchsia-red to bright white at the tip and a mildly spicy flavor. It helps transform insecurities into a deep appreciation for self.

Japanese Wasabi Radish

This daikon-type radish is spring green with a white interior that delivers a tingling wasabi flavor. It supports you in releasing what is no longer valuable, be that possessions, relationships, or aspects of yourself.

Purple Plum Radish

With its stunning purple skin, radiant white interior, and sweet flavor, the purple plum radish supports clarity and vividness in dreams.

White Hailstone Radish

A white spring radish with a very mild taste, the white hailstone radish brings a sense of joy, light, and freedom to conversation and engagement with others.

Zlata Radish

Zlata means "gold" in Czech, and indeed, this spicy variety looks like a sphere of pale gold. It brightens the intellect by pushing back emotional interferences and organizing thoughts and in this way supports analytical thinking.

❦ Squash Varieties

Acorn Squash

Acorn squash supports the maturing of the female principle in both men and women, a metamorphosis that brings about the qualities of inner strength, nurturing sensitivity, and loving wisdom that is not emotionally dependent. It is helpful in seeding the feminine aspect in humanity.

Butternut Squash

Butternut squash heals loss of a balanced perspective, which can lead to being overly internalized and demanding, and concentrating on yourself and what you have or haven't got.

Delicata Squash

Delicata brings the essence of forgiveness and love. It helps bring back the light and emotional balance after resentment and heavy emotional traumas you can't seem to forget. It is helpful in relationship break-ups and grief/anger obsessive cycles.

Kabocha Squash

This sweet-tasting squash promotes moving through the world with a sense of safety and confidence. It helps you to develop a sense of exhilaration while exploring life.

Yellow Crookneck Squash

This variety heals your aversion to routine and structure in daily life.

Zucchini Squash

Zucchini matures the male/yang principle in both men and women and promotes positive creativity that in turn nurtures an awareness of the needs of the environment while achieving your goals. It is helpful in balancing achievement with life-sustaining qualities such as caring and protecting the community and family spirit.

❧ *Tomato Varieties*

Beefsteak Tomato

This variety is deeply fortifying to the emotional body, bringing robustness to the sensations you experience.

Black Krim Tomato

This tomato helps heal deep depression that is debilitating.

Brandywine Pink Tomato

Brandywine allows the energy of love to penetrate into every cell and into all manifestations of your being.

> The French call tomatoes *pommes d'amour,* "apples of love." The Italians affectionately name them "golden apples." When they worked their way from Central and South America to Europe in the sixteenth century, controversy surrounded this fruit/vegetable. They might be fatal. They might be an aphrodisiac. No one knew, but one thing was certain: they were too intriguing to ignore. That our ancestors took a risk, survived, and created fantastic tomato recipes is homage to the siren-like powers of this plant. The tomato has continued to shake things up: it is scientifically a fruit (*Solanum lycopersicum* is the berry of a plant from the nightshade family) but is also considered a vegetable in cooking due to its savory preparation.

Cherokee Purple Tomato

This variety helps heal the separation between the heart and the mind, allowing both to work in tandem.

Cherry Tomato, Black Cherry

Black Cherry tomato helps clear the energy of past sexual relationships you no longer want in your continuum.

Cherry Tomato, Sunrise Bumble Bee

This variety helps balance conditional and addictive patterns of loving and facilitates understanding that relationships are powerful catalysts for learning and growth; it allows you to stay in process while whatever lesson being offered is learned.

Green Zebra Tomato

Green Zebra tomato teaches you how to cultivate yourself and release the restrictions of artificial rules and limits imposed on you, allowing you to tap into your deep creativity and tend to the aspects of life you want to nurture inside and out.

Hillbilly Tomato

This tomato promotes trust, openness, and a renewed interest in life, allowing the heart to open after experiencing conflict.

Pantano Romanesco Tomato

This variety helps heal a shattered heart.

Valencia Tomato

Valencia gently opens your heart, allowing the release of fear and pain stored in your subconscious and cellular memory, thus restoring your innate innocence.

FRUITS

From a botanical standpoint, a fruit is the mature or ripened ovary that contains a flower's seeds. Fruits, in appearance and taste, invoke a juicy abundance that is both natural and sacred. Fruit blossoms in the early spring are a sure sign of nature's rejuvenation, giving joy and hope to all. The fruit has long been associated with the feminine principle of fecundity and abundance, associated with goddesses of fruitfulness, plenty, and the harvest. Fruits are sensual and sticky and are commonly used to describe aspects of eroticism. Parents often admonish their children to eat their vegetables. Fruit, associated with pleasure, requires no cajoling to enter her garden gates.

> *Women are peonies, spring flowers, lotuses and bowers.*
> *Women are pomegranates, peaches, melons and pearls.*
> *Women are receptacles, crucibles,*
> *vessels and worlds.*
> *Women are the fruit of life, the*
> *nourishing force of Nature.*
>
> Yuan-Shih Yeh-Ting Chi, Tao Tsung-I,
> in Margo Anand's *The Art of Sexual Ecstasy*

Apple (General)

Apple gives rise to greater understanding of oneself and the environment by accessing the unfolding but unused aspects of the self. It connects the conscious and unconscious mind for growth and deepens the creative impulse that leads to beauty here on Earth. When cut through lengthwise, an apple reveals a near perfect pentagram, or five-pointed star, with each point containing a seed, which supports understanding of the tenet "As above, so below," or the microcosmic-macrocosmic principle. See specific apple varieties beginning on page 61.

The apple is one of the most varied fruit species on the planet, with more than 7,500 varieties.

Apricot

This downy, yellowish, sometimes rosy fruit brings balance and stabilizes mood swings and extreme emotional states. It promotes an exchange between the mental and subtle bodies, facilitates the reconciliation of internal conflicts and strong negative emotions that have been stored in the body, and empowers you to take responsibility for your life and make the changes necessary for health and well-being, thus fostering delight in life itself.

Avocado

This versatile stone fruit with a creamy texture harmonizes the body and mind by dissolving emotional tension and the negative influence of past pain that can cause you to turn inward and harden against love offered. It offers shelter when you are feeling overwhelmed with emotion, allows you to become more vulnerable to others without feeling fear, and facilitates intimacy and healing through touch.

Banana

This phallic fruit helps you understand the role of sexuality and how male and female energies are intertwined on the subtle level, making it helpful for those exploring the concept of divine marriage as described in alchemical texts and delving into higher sexual practices like tantra with a partner.

Berry (General)

Energetically, berries refine the feminine principle, bringing joy, beauty, and grace. A berry, by definition, is "a small roundish juicy fruit without a stone," although one could argue that a berry is "a celebration for the mouth." See specific berry varieties beginning on page 65.

Caper

The fruit of the caper bush, consumed pickled and salted, helps balance mood swings and stabilizes the emotions.

Cherry

The old song "Life Is Just a Bowl of Cherries" gives meaning to this fruit's energetic properties: for authentically being happy to be who you are and celebrating all that entails.

Citrus (General)

Citrus is characterized by its distinctive fruit, the hesperidium, which is a berry with the internal fleshy parts divided into segments (typically ten to sixteen) and surrounded by a separable skin. Citrus fruits have a thick, fragrant rind—the essential oils of lemon, lime, bergamot, and orange are produced from the rinds of these fruits—and juicy pulp. Energetically, they bring a zest for living! See specific citrus varieties beginning on page 68.

Coconut

Coconut promotes endurance and perseverance for completing tasks, which in turn helps you manifest your full potential; it provides strong, steady energy and the ability to welcome challenges and be solution-oriented.

> Botanically speaking, the coconut is considered a fibrous, one-seeded drupe, also known as a dry drupe. Loosely defined, it is a fruit, a nut, and a seed.

Date

This fruit opens your eyes to seeing and feeling life as a lover, the way ecstatic poets like Rumi and Hafiz experienced life itself as a lover. This allows you to embrace life in all of its aspects, extending yourself joyfully and participating fully in what life offers you.

Dragon Fruit/Pitaya

This dazzling fruit is the product of a night-blooming cactus commonly known as pitaya or moonflower. It offers an invitation to enter the "Garden of Earthy Delights," a place where you can play with magic and delight here on Earth, opening you to experiencing enchantment, amusement, and discoveries that fascinate, astonish, and bring wonderment.

Fig

Fig opens the higher channels of the mind and decoding the memory of your deepest origins to reveal the inner fruit and nectar that's stored in your soul. You in essence become the alchemical holy vessel, gaining access to your deepest knowing and essence.

Grape

This luscious fruit brings soulfulness, the expression of incredible depth that provides softness toward the human experience. It is not the quest for perfection, but instead the practice of exploring what it means to be fully human. It is growing to love the seemingly disorderly and paradoxical aspects of human incarnation and staying within that process without shutting down, until the rich gift of experience has bloomed.

Guava

Guava balances the emotions and cleans the heart chakra, easing tension and anger stuck in the energetic heart. It improves personal expression, confidence, creativity, and love of beauty and the arts.

Kiwi Fruit

Kiwi alerts you that either your muse has arrived or that you need to summon your muse. It tells you there's a spark of creative fire within your higher imagination that's available to you, and you should follow this energy now, while it's available. Muse energy can be subtle, fleeting, and tricky to understand, but always worth the effort.

Mango

Mango promotes sexual bonding and the ability to put into action what you're feeling in your heart. It stirs the energy of desire and passion and couples it with an eagerness to bond and create with another, ultimately allowing a couple to share beautiful, helpful energies.

Melon (General)

Frost-tender annuals with soft, hairy, trailing stems and clasping tendrils, melons bear large round-to-lobed leaves and yellow unisexual flowers. Botanically, the fruits are a type of berry known as a pepo, and they vary greatly in size, shape, surface texture, and flesh color and flavor, depending on the variety. Energetically, they bring the refreshing energy of fairness, truth, and integrity. See specific melon varieties beginning on page 70.

Nectarine

Nectarine helps seal the cracks in your cosmic vessel so that you can soothe your soul and revitalize your life force.

Olive

The olive opens you to the frequency of bringing profound knowledge into conscious awareness for practical use. This stone fruit teaches creative visualization and how to harness natural laws so that you can manifest your ideas in the world for practical ends. You can use this energy for finding the right actions to bring about intended results. Olive vibrates to the archetype of Athena.

Papaya

Papaya aids in spiritualizing the emotions, especially the loving energies that connect you to another person. It aligns the energies of the second chakra with those of the heart and crown chakras.

Passion Fruit

Passion fruit helps you remember that your truest mission is to reflect the dormant divinity within your being, allowing you to be a living mediator between heaven and earth, so that the budding passion of the soul can be understood and realized.

"I call the light and high aspects of my being *spirit,* and the dark and heavy aspects *soul.* Soul is at home in the deep, shaded valleys. Heavy, torpid flowers saturated with black grow there. The rivers flow like warm syrup. They empty into huge oceans of soul. Spirit is a land of high white peaks and glittering jewel-like lakes and flowers. Life is sparse and sounds travel great distances. There is soul music, soul food, and soul love. People need to climb the mountain not simply because it is there, but because the soulful divinity needs to be mated with the spirit."

HIS HOLINESS THE 14TH DALAI LAMA

Peach

Peach vibrates to the energy of the muses, the goddesses of the arts, and helps incite the gift of art in all expressions. The precious gift of peach is to open you to the memory of the muse in your own heart and the joyous expression that flows from this wellspring.

Pear

Pear empowers you to bring the highest spiritual energy into the material realm and teaches you how to use this energy to find practical solutions to problems. It increases the awareness and effective use of personal power.

Persimmon, Fuyu

Persimmon facilitates sinking into the intuitive root of your being to ground subtle knowing. It unseals the female receptive principle and opens you quietly to the moon energy in daily life, to experiencing the blissful power of deep seeing, understanding, feeling, and sensuality.

Absorbing energies without being rooted can bring about a state of denseness and disassociation, where you feel fearful, scattered, and nervous, pushing or trying but feeling inadequate. Persimmon helps counter this.

Pineapple

Pineapple brings joy, playfulness, communion, and bonding among friends and opens the heart to kindness, gratitude, and playfulness. It brings out childlike qualities, alleviates stress, and encourages wonderment, honesty, availability, openness, and finding commonality. If you feel like you're locked in a humdrum routine and don't see the magic and beauty of life all around you, this fruit contradicts that heaviness, adding sparkle to everyday experiences.

Plantain

Plantain helps shift sexual difficulties caused by incorrect sexual self-image, which is often adopted in the early, formative years.

Plum

Teaching self-love, self-esteem, and trust, plum offers dynamic support when you're struggling with self-doubt, unable to appreciate your true worth, and underestimating yourself. It brings openmindedness and teaches boldness to those who are reserved and shy by nature.

Pluot

Pluots are a hybrid between the Japanese plum, *Prunus salicina*, and the apricot, *Prunus armeniaca*.

Eating a pluot is an invitation into the depths of the dark waters of the unconscious. This allows you to see the world with your eyes closed, a very internal perspective and an exceptional state for meditation, prayer, chanting, and any form of stillness where you want to explore the profundity of creation. From these fecund waters, the conscious world is born. Use pluot when you want to explore the realm of archetypes and their impact on human evolution—your evolution—and how to harness the energy of these archetypes for dynamic personal growth, which will bring results that defy what the linear mind can grasp.

Pomegranate

I owe much to this fruit, being one of my major plant allies for navigating my interior life in conjunction with my exterior life. Pomegranate is the fruit of Persephone, daughter of Zeus and Demeter and queen of the underworld and the personification of vegetation and the season of spring. This fruit has a tough exterior, containing off-white membranes (the Kore, or maiden aspect of Persephone); these cradle vibrant, individually "wrapped" purple or red seeds, which are difficult to access (her queen of the underworld aspect). This fruit is a clear example of the doctrine of signatures, meaning the way a plant looks helps explain its function. Consuming this fruit allows you—not unlike Persephone—to divide your energy in a balanced way between the two realms, your personal interior life that only belongs to you, and your expression of yourself out in the world. The underworld is a very soulful place, where fertility begins, and where the goddess lived as queen for part of the year, nurturing fertility. The other part of the year she lived aboveground in her role as Kore, the maiden, where she personified spring, when her latent interior expression came into bloom. In this expression of self, as with the vibration of pomegranate, you can grow anything: relationships, family, inner work, artistic expression, and so on.

Pomelo/Pummelo

Pomelo assists those with latent teaching abilities, allowing this gift to blossom. This may express itself through writing, teaching in a classroom setting, or working with students one-on-one.

Prickly Pear

It is as it is.

Unknown

The tuna, or fruit, of the paddle cactus allows you to stay centered and act out of a sense of inner calmness, taking a breath and assessing a situation rather than getting angry about things that have happened and circumstances you cannot change in the present.

Quince

This fruit is a master healer that brings expansive love and regeneration while easing depression and lethargy. It supports alignment with higher spiritual visions, amplifies positive thought forms, and is a great balancer of the heart chakra. It also simulates regeneration of the energetic body and floods the physical body with the vibration of enlightenment.

Star Fruit

This well-named fruit connects you to the starry realms, and if you have an incarnation pattern that vibrates to being a child of the stars, it helps you remember your celestial roots and ground this knowledge in your daily life for the betterment of others. It also creates a buffer for you so that learning to navigate life on Earth is not so harsh.

Tamarind

Tamarind strengthens your ability to act decisively from a clear sense of what you want and who you are.

❧ *Apple Varieties*

Ambrosia Apple

Ambrosia promotes opening up your "inner hearing," providing clarity so that you can respond to what needs to be acknowledged.

Ananas Reinette Apple

This variety sweetens the troubled mind when you're anxious about your abilities and their execution.

Belle de Boskoop Apple

Belle de Boskoop provides relief from the intensity of your fears by allowing them to be released in an opalescent energy, and holding space for you while you process those energies.

Black Gilliflower Apple

This apple supports deep transformation, allowing you to address core issues and remold their energy, releasing you from these ingrained patterns.

Braeburn Apple

This apple provides protection and sanctuary from negative energies, allowing the subtle body to filter them out.

> The Braeburn apple was first discovered growing in the Braeburn Orchard in New Zealand in 1952. It was a chance seedling, meaning it was not bred intentionally but was created by nature.

Cosmic Crisp Apple

This variety offers a subtle sharpening and refining of your conscious awareness, expanding your ability to perceive in new ways.

D'Arcy Spice Apple

D'Arcy Spice apple promotes forgiveness and softening of the heart.

Esopus Spitzenburg Apple

This apple helps you clearly communicate deeply held beliefs from a place of strength.

> Thomas Jefferson grew the Esopus Spitzenburg apple at Monticello, and it is said to have been one of his favorite apples.

Fuji Apple

Fuji apple brings calm and quiet to an overactive mind, helping you achieve peaceful tranquility.

Gala Apple

Gala promotes free-flowing emotional expression and joyful exchange.

Golden Delicious Apple

This variety promotes self-empowerment by strengthening your true nature and helping you filter through emotional experiences so they don't cloud your judgment, causing you to make rash decisions.

Granny Smith Apple

This apple entwines body rhythms with earthly rhythms, creating a beautiful, interlacing flow of energy that connects you to the green mantle—the earth plane, or Mother Earth.

> Granny Smith apples were discovered in Australia in the 1860s, as a chance seedling in a compost pile on the orchard of Maria Ann Smith.

Hidden Rose Apple

This variety opens conduits to other dimensions, thus allowing you access to universal knowledge, and brings the ability to ground this information into your life through your heart.

> The Hidden Rose is so named for its pale green skin and vivid pink flesh.

Honeycrisp Apple

Honeycrisp apple opens you to feminine energies and their mystical aspects; works with your right (intuitive) brain, allowing you to explore the unstructured, magical aspects of the self.

Hudson's Golden Gem Apple

Providing a delicate strength, this apple brings reinforcement to aspects of the self that are tender and in need of protection.

> The original Hudson's Golden Gem was a chance seedling found growing in a fencerow thicket in Oregon and was introduced in 1831 by the Hudson Wholesale Nursery of Tangent, Oregon.

Idared Apple

Idared apple rekindles the flame within by connecting you to the joy of exploring your inner riches.

Lady Apple

Lady apple teaches the art of softness and grace and promotes fluid, elegant physical movements and thoughtful, eloquent speech. It enables you to view the world through kind eyes, leading to magnanimous behavior.

> The Lady apple is thought to be the oldest apple still being grown today, originally from France and dating back to the 1500s.

McIntosh Apple

McIntosh apple assists in overcoming creative blocks by opening the heart and quieting the mind so you can connect with inspiration.

Old Maid in Winter Apple

This variety helps heal the energy around being emotionally malnourished as a child and brings sweet, healing energy, allowing your inner child to thrive.

Opalescent Apple

Opalescent apple helps break the stagnation of making the same mistakes over and over, eases frustration with this process, and supports maintaining the discipline needed to succeed.

Pink Lady Apple

This apple purifies and balances the heart, embodies the energy of the Divine Mother and the Divine Feminine principle, and encourages the heart to gently open, allowing a richer experience of love in the physical body.

Red Delicious Apple

This variety balances spirituality with physical ability, prompting the integration of your higher purpose into daily life. It encourages fulfillment through accepting divine responsibilities.

Snow Apple

Snow apple helps you recognize the principle of wholeness, seeing oneness reflected in all parts of a thing.

Sops of Wine Apple

This apple brings the energy of spontaneity and feeling carefree, allowing you to play.

Winter Banana Apple

This variety helps you express hurt feelings so that others may better recognize your situation and resolution can be had.

Wolf River Apple

By increasing awareness and appreciation for all that's around you this variety brings zest back to living when you're bored.

Yellow Transparent Apple

This apple helps ease the pain around a broken home, including divorce, adoption, or constant bickering you can't escape.

❧ Berry Varieties

Blackberry

Commonly found in the wild as well as being cultivated, this juicy berry heals the compulsion to sacrifice yourself while trying to live up to the expectations of others.

Blackberry, Himalayan

Himalayan blackberry offers strong protection against gossip and what I call "helpful meddling," where someone says or does something that's to your detriment, and indeed causes hurt, but claims it's to benefit you.

Ever hear someone say they're doing or saying something about you, often behind your back, "for your own good"? The fruit of the Himalayan blackberry, considered a noxious weed and an invasive species in some areas of the country, helps you see the truth in such a situation, untangle the knot of confusing energy, and right yourself.

Black Currant

Black currant helps you become still and focused so you can look for answers within instead of rushing around asking questions and seeking counsel from others. It supports you in finding answers in the cave of your own heart.

Blueberry

This berry can help lessen feelings of anxiety and support you in acknowledging and releasing guilt. It enables you to honestly own the true cause of your thoughts and actions and release blame, either of yourself or others, ultimately allowing healing.

Cloudberry

A wild plant found in the northern regions, cloudberry helps you see the indestructible light of purity that resides deep within.

Cranberry

Cranberry promotes inner discipline and stimulates the right balance of flexibility and restraint.

Elderberry

This medicinal berry is toxic when taken raw, so elderberry must be cooked or dried before being consumed.

Elderberry opens you to receiving the spiritual energy that is all around us and to be taught by this energy. This is an intimate, one-on-one type of learning, lessons the Divine specifically has tailored for you.

Goji Berry

This Asian native, usually eaten dried, like a raisin, is helpful for studying ancient wisdom traditions like Buddhism, Vedanta, Taoism, and so on.

Gooseberry

This berry helps you move toward emotional balance when you are depressed and strengthens the psyche so that you can develop enthusiasm for life, especially after experiencing loss or illness, where it helps release associated fears.

Huckleberry

This traditional food of First Nations peoples supports you in taking ideas and visions and turning them into reality, acting in the right moment in the right way, allowing you to hit your mark, doing exactly that which brings the intended results.

"I'm your huckleberry" is an old-timey way of saying that you're precisely the right person for a specific job, or "I'm your man" in modern parlance. The quote is famously attributed to Doc Holliday in the movie *Tombstone*.

Marionberry

This cultivar of the blackberry helps heal the deep yearning that shackles you due to desiring the unattainable.

Raspberry

Raspberry offers shelter if you're an empath who identifies with the emotions and other energetic states of those around you to an uncomfortable extent. It helps enclose your aura and creates energetic boundaries to separate you from others' extremes so you can enjoy only the exchanges you wish to engage in.

Strawberry

Strawberry encourages being adventurous and daring and willing to take a risk and stretch for things out of your reach and getting them. It facilitates going headfirst and trusting the Divine to deliver and offers wonderful encouragement to venture out of your known environment and experience the wonders of the world and its treasures.

> Strawberry gets its name from an Anglo-Saxon word meaning "spreading berry," due to its abundant, sprawling shoots that grow out from the mother plant.

❦ Citrus Varieties

Bergamot

> The rind of bergamot contains a large amount of essential oil. It is this oil or the dried bergamot peel that produces Earl Grey tea's characteristic floral-citrus taste. The sour flesh is rarely eaten alone but shines in curds and marmalades; the zest is often used in pastries and other sweet confections.

Bergamot helps you value simplicity and overcome the tendency to try too hard or think too much, which can make things more complex than they need to be. Resting in simplicity helps to develop a sunny outlook, feelings of contentment, and serenity.

Blood Orange

Blood orange teaches you how to share your gifts and talents, allowing your natural charisma to shine forth.

Citron/Buddha's Hand

> The Buddha's hand is unique in that it has little juice or pulp. Instead it is used for its rind, which has a sweet, lemon-blossom aroma with a mild-tasting pith that is not bitter. Most often candied and used in baking or as a sweet, it can also be zested or shaved thinly as a unique topping for fish, tofu, or salads. It is a stellar ingredient for a light vinaigrette.

This citrus helps you question your reality, ask the hard questions, pull back the curtains of your life, and start your own unique journey to uncover the truths that are tailor-made for you.

Common Orange

Orange brings out your hidden desires and dissolves frustration and low self-esteem, allowing you to bask in the warm glow of happiness.

Grapefruit

Grapefruit is helpful for when you are trapped in the authoritarian powers of others and cannot figure out how to break free. It will help you dissolve those bonds and find the energy to move forward into a more supportive environment.

Kumquat

Kumquat moves you toward honest, meaningful connections with people, allowing you to feel into the frustration that arises when you're ensnared in shallow, empty, or obligatory relationships, teaching you how to shift this stuck energy by seeking greater depth in yourself and in other people. Ultimately it allows you to get past protective facades.

Lemon

Lemon is of two minds, both very valuable. On one hand, it dispels darkness through merriment. Gaiety is the means to purify that which shackles your joy. Lemon dissolves this in ripples of laughter. On the other hand, this fruit teaches fulfillment in finding nourishment from a spiritual source that brings inner security and joy. Goals and desires are reached, and this brings a sense of completion and satisfaction. Lemon accomplishes this by helping you gather all of your energy and intellectual focus and then directing it toward your intended goal or desire.

Lemon really does teach that laughter is the best medicine.

Lime

This fruit brings out the gifts of joy, emotional clarity, and inner sparkle and helps shift you out of resentfulness, contraction, apathy, and irrationality.

Mandarin Orange

This citrus aids in inner-child work, allowing you to work with deep-seated fears while latent abilities are brought to the surface. It permits you to see how you are perceived by others, thus allowing you to see yourself more clearly so that difficulties and struggles can be viewed in a clear light. It is supportive in counseling situations when you are working with deep emotions, feelings, childhood memories, and associated bodily sensations.

Tangerine

Tangerine helps you grow into adulthood when there's been a habitual pattern (either self-directed or having been forced on you) of staying in a child's energy, such as with the Peter Pan syndrome.

❦ Melon Varieties

Cantaloupe

Cantaloupe teaches the concept of accepting the shadow side of those you love (or have close bonds with), which is a natural part of being human, and how important it is to allow others their own time to process and work with whatever energy they are struggling with in order to bring about true change.

Honeydew Melon

Honeydew teaches humor and equanimity, the ability to laugh at yourself and not make mountains out of molehills.

Watermelon

Watermelon fosters positive self-esteem and allows you to see the beauty of your life, and not just focus on what you would like to shift; this allows you to rest in the sweetness of the present moment.

WILDCRAFTED PLANTS AND EDIBLE FLOWERS

Wildcrafting is a precious act. Seeing and feeling into the landscape where you pluck a flower or trim cedar leaves and observing how the plants live and grow helps you tap into their energy.

It is best practice to ask the plants for permission to harvest them. While everybody will communicate with plant life differently, here is my process:

- I do a short meditation to help me connect. Feeling my feet planted firmly in the ground, I envision myself growing roots, becoming part of the surrounding environment. With my right hand on my heart and my left hand on my stomach, I let my breath and body rhythms synchronize with the sounds around me—the wind, the leaves, the birds. When I feel connected to the environment, I make my inquiry.
- Hovering my left hand over the plant, I ask, "May I harvest you?" (I honestly chat up the plant. Just say what is in your heart and what comes to mind; real dialogue is helpful. If I am engaging with an especially chatty plant, thoughts will fill my mind.)
- If I feel a cold tingling, I know that is a "yes." If I feel heat, for me that is a "no."
- If I get a yes, I like to leave an offering as a thank-you and as a way to bond. Tobacco was traditionally used as an offering, but any gift from the heart works—you might use a seashell, a beautiful stone, or even a strand of your own hair. Most plants also like to be tenderly stroked before you leave.

Before wildcrafting, or foraging, please educate yourself: research what plants in your area are endangered, threatened, and sensitive species, and do not harvest those. Watch your step—literally—a misplaced step can harm or kill delicate plants. Overzealous harvesting leads to decline of the plant and harms the health of the ecosystem. Be especially considerate of or avoid harvesting slow-growing plants. Continually look for new places to harvest so that areas can rest and rejuvenate. Most places do not require permits when harvesting for personal use on public land, but check the laws in your area, and always ask permission from the landowner to forage on private land.

Borage Flower

The flower of the borage plant enhances your ability to have visions and supports vision quests and journeying. It brings clarity and brightness to the thought process, helps you see your path more clearly, and assists in connecting your inner truth with your newly emerging outer path.

Caper Flower

These pinkish-white edible flower buds, which are usually pickled, bring simplicity.

Carnation Flower Petals

Carnation petals bring a true manifestation of light, allowing it to shine through your heart and mind, letting you radiate love and purity to those around you.

Cedar Leaf Tips and Branches

Cedar is strong medicine and should be used with care, as it contains powerful volatile oils that are toxic if taken in large quantities or for long periods of time. It should not be used during pregnancy or breastfeeding or by those with kidney weakness.

All parts of the cedar tree have traditionally been used by native peoples—leaves, bark, branches, and roots. Soak a plank of cedar wood in water for at least 30 minutes and use on the grill for cooking salmon. A tea of simmered small branches and leaf tips is traditionally used to treat fevers, rheumatic complaints, chest colds, and flu. This brew is enjoyable warm or cold and is easy to make. Simply simmer 2 cups of fresh cedar in 4 cups of boiling water for about 10 minutes until the water becomes a golden color. Strain and sweeten with maple syrup or honey to taste.

Cedar empowers spiritual magnificence. It allows you to experience the lesser qualities of others without giving in to annoyance at their imperfections, enabling you to maintain a strong spiritual center. You become a beacon of light, broadcasting loving majesty and joy, encouraging and inspiring others and attracting those whose own spiritual light has grown dim due to life's difficulties. By standing tall and sharing your majesty of spirit, you can be an inspiration to others, lifting their vibrations and allowing them to develop this strength within themselves.

Chamomile Flower

Chamomile heals overwhelm due to overstimulation, hypersensitivity to the environment, or too much outer activity and sensory congestion.

Dandelion

Everything from the flower down to the roots is edible, but the petals are my favorite part of the dandelion plant. They are wonderful as a garnish or for including in homemade pasta. Combine dandelion petals, turmeric, duck egg, and water and mix with the flour to create your dough. Top with dead nettle pesto (see page 173) for a sumptuous weed-based meal!

Dandelion facilitates the flow of the radiant inner light from a deep place of self-recognition and letting that light shine in all you do. It helps heal ego issues (either too inflated or too diminished), creating a balanced way of navigating the world through a healed and luminous third chakra.

Elderflower

To see a World in a Grain of Sand
And a Heaven in a Wild Flower
Hold Infinity in the palm of your hand
And Eternity in an hour

WILLIAM BLAKE

Elderflower vibrates to nature in all of her vibrant wonder. If you want to understand the miraculous as expressed through the natural world, allowing you to truly see in the way described in William Blake's poem, elderflower is a powerful key for this understanding.

> The blooms of the elder plant are flat-headed sprays of hundreds of tiny, five-petaled, creamy white flowers with prominent stamens. My vibrational essence line Whispering Winds is stabilized in elderflower, as she amplifies all expressions of nature.

Fiddlehead Fern

Fiddlehead opens you to understanding the vibrant serenity of the wilderness, especially the forest floor. It helps you release worldly concerns and be quietly contented with your own light.

Johnny-Jump-Up and Pansy

> Johnny-jump-up, *Viola tricolor,* also known as a wild pansy, is actually a smaller species of pansy; both are in the violet family.

This flower is supportive for sensitive people with a rich inner life who have not incarnated very deeply. It can show you how to join more fully in earthly physical life without sacrificing your sensitivity and refined nature. If so desired, it can teach you how to open your subtle channels between the physical and spirit worlds. This flower can also help those wishing to increase their sensitivity to the unseen realms.

Lilac Flower

Lilacs have a deep-rooted history originating in ancient Greek mythology. It was said that Pan, the god of forests and fields, was hopelessly in love with a nymph named Syringa. One day, as he pursued her through a forest, she became so overwhelmed by his advances that she turned herself into a lilac shrub to disguise herself. To Pan's surprise, he couldn't find Syringa, but he did find the lilac bush, and since a lilac shrub consists of hollow reeds, he cut the reeds and created the first panpipe. The scientific name for lilac is *Syringa vulgaris,* and the name is derived from the Greek word *syrinks,* which means "pipe."

Our culture bases so much of our lives around what we do. We define ourselves through our work and judge our worth based on our outward accomplishments. Pan, or this aspect of lilac, is about being rather than doing, totally surrendering to a bliss that is beyond the mundane. If you're feeling ashamed about any natural sexual impulse, if you are frustrated, bored, agitated, or restless, or if you have an unsatisfying sexual life that doesn't feed your soul, these are all signs that you've been cut off from your deep, natural self. Lilac will help your remember, replenish, and make whole what you've lost. Lilac brings the vibration of the breath of love and sweetness and the energy of spring, youthfulness, and joy. This flower returns you to basics, back to the self, and resets and renews your energy for relationships that lack sweetness.

With both medicinal and culinary applications, lilac's vibrant lavender-to-magenta color and heady, aromatic scent depict the vibrational action of the flower: it brings the energy of soulfulness and passion. In the throes of a sexual experience with the right partner, a person loses their world identity, and other than death or religious and spiritual ecstasy it's the only time when we truly let ourselves go completely. A sense of oneness is experienced. The essence of lilac connects you to your raw, natural self, deeply melding you with nature, profound bliss, divine play, true surrender, and the use of sexuality as an ecstatic gateway to the Divine.

You may have noticed that in Greek mythology nymphs are always turning into plants to avoid some god or goddess. This should not be read as violence, as archetypal language is complex and symbolic. It's more along the lines that we as mortals often do not fare well in the raw energy of the Divine, and these plants are the emissaries of the gods and goddesses that allow us to touch an aspect of their divinity without being overwhelmed.

Marigold Flower

Marigold's brilliant golden blooms spiritualize the intellect, enhance willpower and mental clarity, and attune you to the sun.

Nasturtium Flower

This piquant bloom is excellent for entering endless expansion while maintaining your center and savoring life experiences. It encourages you to live life fully and consciously.

Nasturtium Leaf

Nasturtium leaf has a mild peppery flavor with an aroma reminiscent of mustard. It helps ease stressed, overextended states. If you are facing too many demands and taking on other people's "stuff," this leaf helps you communicate boundaries and set limits with humor and ease.

Nettle, Purple Dead

This plant calms emotions so you can speak without fear, allowing words to come from the deepest levels of the self. It is helpful not only for difficult conversations but also for public speaking and for writing.

Red or purple dead nettle is distinguished from stinging nettle by its dark purple flowers and the fact that, unlike its cousin the stinging nettle, it doesn't sting, hence it is "dead."

Nettle, Stinging

> *Tender-handed stroke a nettle,*
> *And it stings you for your pains,*
> *Grasp it like a man of mettle,*
> *And soft as silk remains.*
>
> AARON HILL, SCOTTISH POET (1685–1750)

Turn to stinging nettle when you are at a crossroads and need to be aware of choices that are seemingly hidden from view to inform your decision-making. This allows you to channel your energy in a new direction.

Purslane

One of the least-appreciated edible weeds, purslane's energy is to align the base chakra with the brow chakra (the third eye), linking understanding with higher purpose.

Queen Anne's Lace

Queen Anne's lace is good for integrating information from past lessons and experiences into present-time awareness and for accessing eternal wisdom from nature.

Red Clover

Red clover clears being overly swayed by the opinions of others and caught up in mass hysteria or negativity and instead brings steadfast hope and optimism.

Rose Hip

Rose hip promotes inner radiance and enhances the state of joy between those in a relationship. This is often achieved by bringing up old issues and patterns between people to be dealt with and cleared, allowing a couple to move forward with a clean slate.

Rose Petal

Rose stimulates the desire to work toward enlightenment via the path of the heart. With love being the key to unfolding the path at each stage of development, this is a route filled with grace that teaches strength in gentleness, which results in harmonious actions. It's a very good flower to use if you don't want to attend the school of hard knocks along the way.

Saint-John's-Wort

This plant helps clear nocturnal fears, nightmares, restless sleep, the energy around childhood bed-wetting, and discordant energy around the relationship with the father.

Violet

Violet opens you up to working with the fairy realm. She is not very chatty at first and speaks in subtle ways, in signs, dreams, and whispers. She often requires a long courtship to know her magic.

FINISHING SALTS

In the beginning—our beginnings—Earth was a watery planet, completely enveloped in a salty primordial ocean. Our bodies still benefit from, and indeed crave, salts that have not been super-heated, processed, and treated—drastic steps that remove the precise electrolytes, trace minerals, and elements our bodies desire. Salt that has been processed is approximately 99 percent sodium chloride—so, unfortunately, missing much of the health-giving properties of the primordial ocean from which all life on Earth arose.

Finishing salts are not used during the cooking process but sprinkled sparingly after the dish is finished. Less is more in this context, as these salts have complex flavor profiles.

Fleur de Sel

This salt, whose name means "flower of salt" in French, is harvested in the traditional, labor-intensive way, passing seawater through a network of dikes and ponds and then harvesting the purest, whitest layer off the top. The fine crystals are rich in minerals and offer a silken texture with a delicate taste that has just the faintest hint of brine. Fleur de sel brings refinement to life, helping you appreciate beauty such as that found in ballet, symphony, opera, and other classical arts. It stimulates a hunger to try new things, which might manifest as being a tourist in your own town—trying new restaurants, visiting museums you never seem to find time for, or joining a salon whose pure purpose is the discussion of ideas for the joy of it.

Himalayan Pink Salt

This 250-million-year-old, Jurassic-era pink sea salt, known for its healing properties, is a pure, hand-mined salt found deep within the pristine foothills of the Himalayan mountains. Believed to stimulate circulation and remove toxins such as heavy metals from the body, it has been used for centuries in folk remedies. The energy of this salt is the power of three: the undivided primal waters, the wisdom energy of intuition, and the power of logic operating through you. The *undivided primal waters* are pure potentiality, the "all thing" before taking form. *Intuition* is a knowing that is felt and understood in an amorphous way. This energy is sometimes described as a fire of knowing, or testimony to a truth that cannot be proven or even articulated but is so powerful that it shapes lives and destinies. *Logic* can be understood as the expression of your intuition, dropped into form at a vibration dense enough that the human mind can begin to organize, process, and utilize the divine information being expressed and act upon it.

Kilauea Onyx Sea Salt

This Hawaiian sea salt has a deep obsidian black color and moist, silky texture. It is solar evaporated with purified black lava rock to add minerals, then combined with activated charcoal to add detoxifying effects. The energy of this salt invites you into the womb of self, a portal to dreamtime. Entering into silence within, you will find deep rest and introspection within this hallowed space. Here you can dream into being the next turn of the wheel to be co-created with the Divine. Contrariwise, if you become lost in the labyrinth of self—which might present as malaise, becoming tangled in your thoughts and unable to find solutions, or self-created isolation that is to your detriment—this salt can act as a midwife and support your return to the light.

Molokai Red Sea Salt

This Hawaiian sea salt is solar evaporated and combined with red volcanic clay, or *alaea,* to achieve an ultra-mineral-rich sea salt with the pristine energy of deep Pacific waters. Hawaiians believe that the baked alaea clay, which is composed of more than eighty minerals, provides a variety of benefits, with detoxifying and healing powers. Historically, this salt has also been used for ceremonial purposes such as blessing and purifying seagoing canoes. This salt cleanses and purifies, helping to dispel heavy or dark energy that can overshadow life and allowing sunshine and deep radiance to fill your being once again.

HERBS AND SPICES

Spices are plants used to flavor foods that come from the root, stem, seed, fruit, or flower of a plant, whereas herbs come from the leafy green part of a plant. Energetically, herbs and spices bring diversity and flavor to life, making it interesting!

Allspice

Allspice brings strength and balance to the third chakra and helps you manifest your will on the material plane from a place of integrity.

Asafoetida

Asafoetida helps you integrate information when you're overwhelmed with the rate at which it is coming in.

Basil

Basil bridges the mundane and the Divine to foster love of all types, as well as forgiveness and compassion.

Bay Leaf

Deeply energizing for the subtle body, bay leaf clears blocked or stagnant energies and renews vitality and energy flow.

Black Pepper

Black pepper promotes living by your personal code of conduct and supports being precise and a specialist in whatever endeavor you're currently exploring.

Caraway Seed

This spice supports letting down your defenses and allowing others to get close to you.

Cardamom

Cardamom fosters feelings of contentment regardless of outside circumstances.

Celery Seed

Celery seed increases devic communication and your "green thumb" abilities and encourages you to prepare nutritious meals.

Chicory Root

Chciory root eases possessiveness and the need to control and manipulate people and situations. This often occurs because you feel unloved for your own special qualities and fear you won't get enough without manipulating. This spice awakens the quality of selfless service and unconditional love, allowing you to draw from your own source of divine energy rather than taking it from others.

Chive

Chive helps quiet the mind, bringing peace and detachment from repetitive thoughts.

Cilantro Leaf

Cilantro helps balance poor internal anchoring and being overly affected by environmental factors.

Cinnamon

This dynamic spice helps to pull you from the mire of self-defeat, self-pity, self-destruction, and not taking care of yourself. By holding space for you, when no one else seems to want to and it feels as if the whole world is against you, cinnamon helps you explore the energy of negative self-fulfilling prophecies and shift the energy before they come to be. We all get down sometimes, and this spice helps you properly explore your gloomy feelings so that you can be done with them.

Clove

Clove deepens the creative impulse.

Coriander

Coriander brings a sparkling effervescence to your emotional body and demeanor.

Cubeb

Cubeb heals "hot" issues like anger, quarrelsomeness, and confrontational behavior.

Cumin

Cumin helps heal feelings in your body of being uneasy and not enjoying the sensual pleasures of being on this Earth.

Dill

Dill alerts you to the need for change and growth and helps clarify the energetic roots of an illness that's been festering away and needs to come to a head so that cleansing and new growth can occur.

Fennel Seed

This spice offers upliftment from drudgery for those times when you are duty-bound and obligated to work in ways and on tasks that you abhor, that are not in alignment with your nature but you must finish. Fennel seed offsets this by helping you find a measure of enjoyment or pride in what you're doing and seeing its value.

Fenugreek

Fenugreek promotes freedom from attachments—such as outdated, dogmatic, and emotional beliefs—that may hinder your life.

Filé Powder

This spice helps remove the paradigm of having no expression of personal choice.

Galangal

Galangal supports alignment with synchronistic events and grace.

Ginger Root

Ginger root cultivates the attitude of having no fear of criticism, and instead standing tall and basking in the glory of who you truly are.

Grains of Paradise

This spice helps us remember that we co-create with the Divine to bring our visions into reality.

Horseradish

Horseradish ushers in the energy of the Divine Masculine, being a protector and champion for others and yourself.

Juniper Berry

Juniper opens you to spiritual gifts such as clairvoyance, clairaudience, and being a clear channel—all information beyond the rational mind.

Juniper berries are not technically a berry but are actually the female seed cone of the juniper tree. They have a long history of medicinal and culinary use (including as flavoring in gin), and juniper tea was once used as a disinfectant for surgeons' tools.

Kaffir Lime Leaf

Good for energetic protection and cord cutting, kaffir lime leaf supports liberation from limiting thoughts and behavioral patterns.

Lemongrass

Lemongrass helps heal the lack of self-control and volatile expressions of oneself.

Mace

Mace helps heal shock that occurs at the solar plexus that leaves you feeling panicked, as in thoughts like *I'm not good enough* or *I'm not capable.* It fortifies you so you're willing to try.

Marjoram

Marjoram brings the energy of *hygge*—a coziness and comfortable conviviality with feelings of wellness and contentment. Its energy is a warm embrace, the perfect cup of tea, sitting by the fire with a book, a soft pillow, a warm bowl of soup, and so on. Use marjoram in times when you are in need of comfort and being held and uplifted on an emotional level. English botanist John Gerard (1545–1612) recommended it "for those who are given to over-much sighing."* Traditionally it has also been used to help curb excessive sexual impulses.

Mint

Mint helps those who are introverted open up to the world and recognize divine timing concerning when to share and when to retreat.

---

*Tisserand, *Art of Aromatherapy,* 252.

Mustard Seed

Mustard seed helps you connect to and address deep karmic issues that surface for resolution, and keeps your focus on what needs to be done in the moment to make changes.

Nutmeg

Nutmeg supports abstract understanding and dreaming and visualizing what could be.

Oregano

Oregano helps shift laziness, bargaining, and pay-offs to gain advantages for yourself for loving because of a need for domination or gain to a healthier place of standing firm in your center and providing for yourself and others from a place of strength and true affection.

Paprika

Paprika cultivates the ability to initiate projects on every level with passion, enthusiasm, and warmth.

Parsley

Parsley fosters forgiveness and the resolution of conflict.

Peppermint

Peppermint encourages you to avoid extremes—and in doing so, opens the door to achieving much. It teaches the art of staying in flow/motion when an outcome is impossible to predict, keeping a cool head and observing events unfold with detachment until you see the most auspicious path, and then jumping in with both feet. Peppermint reminds you that life is always in flux and energy can be rechanneled at any given time toward the desired outcome as long you remains poised, present, and cool-minded.

Pink Pepper Seed

This pepper opens you to your erotic, rapturous nature and the feeling of loving being in your body. This gives rise to ecstatic sexuality and supports the healing of shame, body image issues, and frigidity.

Rosemary

Rosemary is for remembrance,
Between us day and night,
Wishing that I might always have
You present in my sight.

FROM WILLIAM HUNNIS,
"A NOSEGAY ALWAYS SWEET"

This herb is a heavy-hitter that teaches you how to wield personal power. It sharpens your intellect, logic, and will and teaches leadership, integrity, courage, self-worth, consciousness, and refinement—and let us not forget remembrance. Rosemary balances the third chakra.

Saffron

Saffron holds the energy of pure consciousness and teaches that when a person is able to raise their energy up to this point, a state of enlightenment is experienced.

Sage

This herb is a master cleanser and purifier that can nullify all discordant energy. This doesn't mean it's permanently removed—you still have to do your personal work to shift the cause of the disharmony—but sage can offer refuge and hold space for you while you do so.

Star Anise

Star anise opens the crown chakra and third eye, helping you see into other realms.

Summer Savory

Summer savory helps release feelings of awkwardness and discomfort and reconnects you to your childlike nature.

Tarragon

Tarragon amplifies your sense of humor and wit and ushers in buoyant, uplifting energy that is infectious.

Thyme

Thyme encourages warmth and receptivity, especially in the use of the spoken word. It teaches you how to use language to heal and creates the energy of inclusiveness and true caring. Thyme helps heal the compulsion to use cutting words, excessive sarcasm, and argumentativeness.

Turmeric

Turmeric supports the transmutation of any situation that doesn't serve your higher self.

Vanilla

Vanilla teaches sensuality, sexual intimacy, and giving and receiving pleasure.

GRAINS

Technically seeds, grains are a remarkable and versatile food source that have continued to be cultivated, uninterrupted, on every continent (except Antarctica) from the most ancient times to the present. No major civilization has ever thrived without growing a basic grain, and each grain has its own legends, traditions, myths, and symbolism. In America we celebrate our "amber waves of grain." The Roman goddess of agriculture, Ceres, presided over the festival of Cerealia, a festival dedicated to all grains. In Egypt Osiris taught humankind how to break up the land following the fertile flooding of the Nile, to sow the seed, and, in due season, to reap the harvest. Energetically, the "staff of life," as grain is known, brings stability and structure.

Barley, Pearl

Barley stimulates the root chakra, which anchors groundedness and an understanding of what abundance means to you such that you can enjoy your earthly experience more. This grain also helps you access past-life and sublimated current-life memories and eases any aggravation around these issues. It can bring awareness to constructive experiences, past or present, where you did something positive and created benefit, and can draw your attention to some event that may have been uncomfortable but helped you learn an important lesson, and the result was valuable to your soul's evolution.

Demeter was known as the Barley Mother, which speaks to this grain's ability to allow you to flower on the earthly plane. Through this plant, the Eleusinian mysteries, the annual initiatory rites held in her honor in ancient Greece, will echo in your current time and space.

Buckwheat

Buckwheat brings a sense of being capable no matter what the task at hand is, allowing you to leverage your inner and outer resources to get the job done. This can involve calling on your own inner knowing, getting help from another person, or learning something new on the fly.

Bulgur Wheat

Bulgur supports major shifts in life and creating a clear path through the maze of fear and confusion by keeping your intuition shining bright, like a guiding star that shows you where you want to go and how to get there.

Farro

Farro promotes loving inclusion of others and positive expectations of goodwill, combined with the ability to trust. It helps erase unfair projection and the expectation of antagonism from others.

Millet

Millet promotes a well-developed sense of individuality balanced with an understanding of how to interact within group dynamics.

Oatmeal

Oatmeal brings a sense of stability, empowerment, and peace in situations where you feel vulnerable or off-balance or just need a reset of energy.

Quinoa

Quinoa promotes holistic thinking and perceiving the physical world and physical life with spiritually clear thoughts so as not to get weighed down by an overly mundane worldview.

Rice (General)

There are more than seven thousand varieties of rice being grown around the world. All require abundant water—during the growing season the plants are submerged in 1 to 8 inches of water. These varied rices form the base for iconic dishes such as jambalaya from the Americas, bibimbap of Korea, paella of Spain, risottos of Italy, sushis of Japan, and the curries of India and Thailand. See specific rice varieties beginning on page 90.

Rye

Rye balances your emotional body while allowing you to stay open to the unfolding of your evolution so that you can accept your rate of growth without judgment.

Teff

Teff is extremely small, taking about 150 seeds to weigh the same as *one* grain of wheat. It is so tiny that the entire grain must be milled; there is no way to remove the germ or the husk. In the Amharic language, *teff* means "lost," because much of the tiny seed disappears when handled and cannot be found if dropped. You may have tried this grain in an Ethiopian restaurant in the delicious injera, a fermented, very sour traditional bread.

This ancient grain of Ethiopia has the capacity to help you understand symbols on many levels, even obscure symbols from past civilizations. This can change your reality when you feel stuck because symbols are frequently a dynamic way for your spiritual helpers to relay information to you.

Wheat, Bread/Hard Red Winter Wheat

Triticum aestivum vulgare, hard red winter wheat, the variety commonly used in bread, brings a deep resonance within the physical form and restores a sense of vitality, leading to action and the ability to move more into life.

Wheat, Durum

Most often used for pasta, this variety of this staple grain opens you to the freedom to love yourself and others and to be open to expressing that love.

❧ Rice Varieties

Arborio Rice

With a high starch content and slightly chewy and sticky consistency, Arborio rice develops a creamy texture when cooked. It helps you develop mandalic or holistic consciousness, synthesizing ideas into a livening wholeness so that you do not see things in bits and pieces but rather as parts of the whole.

Basmati Rice

Long, dry, separate grains with a nutty aroma and flavor, basmati promotes forthright masculine energy and warrior-like spirituality, which confronts and transforms, helping you face challenges head-on without shrinking back.

Brown Rice

The nutritious bran layers are left on brown rice, making it rich in vitamins and minerals and a 100 percent whole-grain food with a chewy texture and a pleasant, slightly nutty flavor. It helps soften your heart and view life from a perspective that encompasses all the possibilities a person can face, therefore losing judgmental attitudes. It helps you realize *one day this could happen to me* and to prepare for the twists and turns that life may present.

Forbidden Rice

Once reserved solely for the Chinese emperor to ensure his health and longevity—and forbidden to anyone else—this is a medium-grain, non-glutinous heirloom rice with a deep purple hue and a nutty, slightly sweet flavor. It helps curb tendencies toward oblivion, which includes any substance used to excess too often, and supports you in finding the strength and desire to anchor into your life without escaping, numbing yourself, or pretending.

Jasmine Rice

Jasmine rice develops a pleasing jasmine aroma while it is cooking, and the moist, soft texture is ideal for soaking up spices and flavors. It helps you release the fear of "doing wrong" and not living up to others' expectations and supports you in finding calm within yourself and listening to your own inner guidance without worry of judgment.

White Rice

With a mild flavor and a light, fluffy texture, white rice encourages serenity and harmony. It realigns and strengthens your energy flow and brings simplicity.

Wild Rice

Wild rice is not related to Asian rice. It's the seed of four species of aquatic grass originally grown by indigenous tribes around the Great Lakes region.

Wild rice teaches the lesson of moving out of the self-imposed bondage of self-centeredness into communion with the larger world. Where you have felt apathetic, angry, jealous, prejudiced, and fearful, you now can see interconnectedness and oneness and thereby sow the energy of harmony and togetherness in every thought and deed.

LEGUMES AND BEANS

Beans and legumes are brimming with soluble fiber and offer tremendous versatility in the kitchen. They are an excellent source of protein and iron and are rich in vitamins, potassium, and calcium and low in fat. Energetically, beans and legumes anchor you in your body and amplify emotional intelligence.

Anasazi Bean

This bean's song is the song of fertility. If you have had a craving for or been drawn to this bean, you are being asked to utilize your unique talents to create fertility in some quadrant of your life. This is a productive time for you that is being divinely supported. Use all of your skills and resources and plant the seeds now so that you can harvest the fruits of your idea and labor in the future.

Anasazi is the Navajo word for "the ancient ones," the cliff-dwelling indigenous peoples who lived in Colorado, New Mexico, Utah, and Arizona around 130 CE. Local legends state that this bean was discovered in the 1900s in the ruins of their dwellings. More likely, Anasazi beans were continuously growing in the American Southwest but had not reached the attention of the broader public.

Black Bean

Black bean brings wild, unbridled energy and energizes any situation (good or bad), as it is an amplifier. When it calls to you, remember to be attentive to your personal energy, environment, and intentions. A great deal of energy is available to you at this time, so make sure it's going where you want it to go!

Black-Eyed Pea

Black-eyed pea asks you to look behind your fears and distinguish what's a healthy concern and what's a projection of past hurts and traumas. If the latter, not to worry—as is the way with the plant kingdom, the vibration of this ally is provided to help you do just that.

Butter Bean

This bean brings the desire to share with others what you deeply love, whatever that may be, with warmth and enthusiasm.

Cannellini Bean

Cannellini offers an invitation to remember your hopes and dreams, things you might have tucked away and almost forgotten due to circumstances, but the seed(s) remain. Now is a good time to water those desires and ponder how you will tend them so as to bring them into reality.

Chickpea/Garbanzo Bean

Sometimes the only way out is through. Difficulties don't vanish just because your mind tells them to. "Energy goes where attention flows" means that actions follow what is uppermost on your mind. It may be necessary to understand the cause of a particular difficulty in order to understand how to resolve it, and to understand why it's not productive to hold on to a problem any longer, as that can create a way of being in the world. Ultimately, we all have to face whatever daunting energy is holding us back, no matter how frightening it is, and move forward anyway. Only then can you allow new outcomes in your life. Chickpea will fortify you and give you the strength to face challenges head-on, with a clear mind and open eyes, ultimately allowing you to resolve the situation at hand.

Edamame

Edamame stimulates sexuality and universal love, and therefore it opens couples to possibilities not yet recognized but just waiting to be activated. This in turn arouses a need to communicate with genuine intimacy. Words alone often fail to communicate the essence of what you are trying to share. Edamame helps you soften, open, and deeply commune. This can be as simple as looking into the eyes of the other person and acknowledging their divinity, a soft touch, a deep embrace, a tender kiss, and awareness of your own body language and what it conveys.

> Edamame allows you to listen gently with mindfulness, to allow your thoughts to form and the words that follow to be prayers you want to share with your beloved.

Fava Bean

> First, "unzip" the fava pod by opening the seam that runs the length of the pod and then remove the beans inside. Blanch the shelled beans for one minute in boiling, salted water; drain and let the beans cool. Pinch the beans to slip off their skins. If the beans are young and fresh, you may not have to skin them.

This exquisitely delicious bean honors the cycle at the end of life and moving into death. No matter how prepared you are, a person's dying process is a devastating time for everyone involved. There are no words to describe the comfort the fava will bring. It may still be difficult and frightening, but fava will open a window to being comforted and ease the fear by helping you connect in the deepest way to the beliefs that have sustained you through life, allowing a deep abiding faith to arise. This is also an excellent bean to use to connect with and celebrate your ancestors.

I frequently spoke with my mother as I wrote this book. She's getting to the age where she has started to consciously think about how she wants to die. We've spent many hours talking about the energy of the fava bean and how she wants her last days to be honored and celebrated. When the time comes close, she wants me cook her a "buttery bowlful of them" (her very words) and simply sit with her holding her hand, telling her stories and listening to hers, and occasionally eating a fava bean.

Flageolet Bean

The flageolet cultivates joy through optimism, living a soulful life, and creating a positive environment filled with beauty. This translates differently for each person, but it's common to want to be surrounded by the sensual aspects of life such as music, food, art, and fragrance.

Gigante Bean

These large white beans, whose name means "giant" in Greek, are very practical: they can help you find the energy and motivation to tidy up loose ends like unpaid bills, sock drawers that runneth over, changing the oil in your car, and so on. Once you clean up the clutter, both physically and mentally, gigante promises you will feel much better.

Kidney Bean

The kidney bean brings understanding and eases worry when you are overwhelmed by remorse and grief over accidents or mistakes made, and it shows the path to reconciliation.

Lentil

The word *lens* comes from the Latin name for the lentil plant. Lentils shine a light and help you see clearly, particularly when you have had too much and need to rein it in or redirect. They support you in understanding how specific subconscious worries are creating energy blocks and impeding the growth of a situation. This is a great plant to ask *What do I need to see?* or *What do I need to recognize?* Loving lentil will remove the scales from your eyes, imparting clarity and understanding of action.

Lima Bean

Lima bean promotes living in a state of wonder, curiosity, and flow.

Lupini Bean

The lupini reminds you to be loving to the people around you and appreciate the simple and beautiful things in life, and that gently engaging with those you care for is just as important as making money or striving toward some goal. It creates balance in your life.

Navy Bean

The navy bean reminds you not to be afraid to take your power, as power has strength, and power is courage. Always use this energy for the benefit of all, as in harvesting the power of nature for good purposes, or carefully respecting the natural world while meeting the real needs of humankind.

Orca Bean/Calypso Bean/Yin-Yang Bean

Living in cooperative balance while moving through cycles is a key gift of this plant. Conception, manifestation, completion and end of the cycle—everything in life moves in cycles and then begins anew. Thoughtful progression through life phases gives personal symbolic meaning to any event. This bean allows you to look at the underlying energy of what's occurring rather than at the event itself. A move, a shift in relationship, a change in work, and so on are all the same at some level in that they express the energy of change. The orca bean allows you to be in harmony within your cycle and glean the gifts at any given point in your journey.

Peanut

Often thought of as a nut, the peanut is actually the seed of the legume plant *Arachis hypogaea*.

Peanuts support the desire to constantly learn by valuing tradition, coupled with the desire for growth and change. They also help you attune to earth energies.

Pinto Bean

Pinto beans teach the art of "plain talk," the ability to be straight in dealing with the truth, combined with the ability to clear up confusion or misunderstanding.

Red Bean

Red beans allow change and chaos to flow through you without you resisting or becoming rigid, helping you flow with situations rather than demand control over them.

NUTS AND SEEDS

Nuts are actually the seeds of plants and most are the seeds of trees. Unlike the seeds we call nuts, culinary seeds come from vegetables (such as pumpkins), flowers (such as sunflowers), and crops grown for a variety of uses (such as flax and hemp). Nuts and seeds promote holistic thinking—perceiving the physical world with spiritually clear thoughts.

Almond

Almond helps arrest the fear of aging and makes the passage of time sacred and not solely experienced through the physical body. It opens you to the complex beauty of the self and a strong inner vitality.

Brazil Nut

This nut reminds you to look at the needs and goals we have in common with others and to seek cooperation and community action rather than attempting to go it alone.

Cashew Nut

Cashew helps hone fine judgment and the ability to discriminate subtle levels of truth, ultimately broadening your viewpoint.

Chestnut

Chestnut aids in clearing your mind of repetitive, unwanted thoughts and restoring serenity and peace of mind that leads to faith, hope, and joy.

> Chestnuts are a seasonal item in most areas, although the brand Galil offers wonderful organic ones that are shelled and ready to eat year-round.

Chia Seed

Chia seed teaches the art of self-sufficiency. It supports you in creating a thriving life built upon the foundation of your own hard work. Chia also teaches the art of tenacity and keeping with your goal, even after setbacks, until you hit the mark.

> *Chia* means "strength" in the Mayan language, and the chia plant certainty lives up to its name. This desert plant is not only drought tolerant, it is known as a "fire following" plant, meaning that it is one of the first to reappear after a devastating wildfire. Remarkably adaptable, chia plants can even self-pollinate if the bees or butterflies don't take care of the job. They will self-sow in the autumn, and they have no known vulnerabilities to pests or diseases.

Cocoa "Bean"

This plant teaches you how to live in joy; useful for those who tend to be bitter and have an over-somber sense of spirituality.

> Originally a native plant of South America, the cacao tree can live up to a hundred years. Its seeds are removed from their pod, fermented for five to seven days, dried (usually in the sun), roasted, ground, and further refined before they become the basis for making chocolate.

Flaxseed

Flaxseed helps promote nonsexual affection between friends.

Hazelnut

Hazelnut fosters the development of skills and supports all form of study, along with the ability to retain useful information.

Hemp Seed

Hemp seed teaches the art of versatility and the ability to wear many hats, so to speak.

Macadamia Nut

Macadamia nut promotes a sunny, serene disposition and counterbalances the energy of being upset easily.

Pecan Nut

Pecan supports the ability to hear and understand your physical body's wisdom.

Pine Nut

Pine nut opens you to profound self-love and self-forgiveness and allows you to experience your emotions in real time versus playing out echoes from the past.

Pistachio Nut

Pistachio opens the heart to a wider spectrum of experience and heightens your intuition for more immediate and sensitive relationships with others.

Poppy Seed

Poppy seed helps you interact with the spirit world and achieve altered states of consciousness.

Pumpkin Seed

See the pumpkin entry on page 33.

Sesame Seed

Sesame balances the third chakra (the solar plexus) and taps into the luminous energy there that is similar to the sun's, strengthening your ability to act decisively from a clear sense of self.

Sunflower Seed

Sunflower helps heal the energy around gender inequality, narcissism, and being cruel or punitive. It teaches valuing a point of view that differs from your own, which can help you open to a radiant emotional life and an understanding of the importance of the emotional body. It fosters the ability to create order and organization, experience moderation and personal discipline, and develop left-brain, dynamic action. Sunflower seed vibrates to the archetype of Apollo and expands appreciation and execution of the classical arts.

DAIRY

Butter and milk are milked from the living cloud; the navel of Order, the ambrosia is born.

RIG-VEDA 9.74.4

I came to my garden, my sister, my bride, I gathered my myrrh with my spice, I ate my honeycomb with my honey, I drank my wine with my milk. Eat, friends, drink, and be drunk with love!

SONG OF SOLOMON 5:1

Milk embodies the soothing energies of a full moon and has been said to offer the gift of soma, the ambrosiac drops of the moon—meaning you should read its energetic gifts archetypally: it is abundant, fertile, soothing, creative, illuminating, nourishing, and fostering and provides wholeness. Ayurvedic physician Dr. David Frawley, director of the American Institute of Vedic Studies, says that milk is of a *sattvic* nature, meaning it promotes the qualities of

> intelligence, virtue and goodness, and creates harmony, balance and stability. It is light (not heavy) and luminous in nature. It possesses an inward and upward motion and brings about the awakening of the soul. Sattva provides happiness and contentment of a lasting nature. It is the principle of clarity, wideness and peace, the force of love that unites all things together.*

One of the primal foods of sattva, pure and unadulterated milk brings peace and calm. Raw milk is also super-rich in healthy bacteria and makes a great probiotic drink that can benefit your digestive system. It has various enzymes that may help improve the digestion of nutrients from other foods. The fat present in raw milk has soluble vitamins including A, K, and E. It is also rich in water-soluble vitamins like C and B complex that are generally destroyed by excessive heat. While the nutritional and energetic qualities will be purer in raw milk, harmful bacteria in unpasteurized dairy products can also cause severe illness. In most areas raw-milk cheese and butter are more easily obtainable than raw milk itself.

The following descriptions apply to milk, whether it's raw or pasteurized and whether it's consumed as milk, cheese, or butter.

Camel Milk

Though one might well imagine that the diet of desert cultures such as the Bedouin relies heavily on camel's milk, it is now available in the United States due to its many health benefits. Energetically, camel's milk brings the energy of caretaking by the archetypal Mother and

---

*Frawley, *Ayurveda and the Mind,* 31.

Father; this succor opens you to being whole, including feelings of unconditional love, trust, hope, healing, fortitude, and resourcefulness. Nurturing such as this brings the gifts of a joyful, loving patience with your process, which allows universal intelligence to direct you to where you need to be while opening you to the full spectrum of experiences in their many colors and shades.

Camel's milk has been consumed by humans for more than six thousand years. Nutritionally, it is richer than cow's milk in vitamins C and B, iron, calcium, magnesium, and potassium. Camels, the living "ships of the desert," exhibit an astonishing ability to produce milk under the harshest of conditions, while also providing transportation, dung for fires, and hair for weaving, profoundly impacting every aspect of life of desert nomadic peoples. In the 1840s, camels were introduced to Australia to aid in the exploration of that country's vast desert outback. There are now thought to be more than 1.2 million of these animals in the wild, which is considered to be the world's largest feral population. Camel milk production has become one of Australia's emerging agricultural industries. The most common species used for this purpose is the dromedary, or Arabian camel, which has one hump.

Cow Milk

> In Sanskrit, every name portends the cosmic meaning of the bearer's relationship to the earth. The cow is called go. Go is also the name for the earth and the holy scriptures. Lord Krishna was called Gopala, the one who protects the cow. "Protecting the cow" is a common, and ancient, expression used to infer the protection of the scriptures, the nurturing of the land, and the celebration of the cow, who is the manifest keeper of the memory of the earth's spiritual dharmas [the law of our nature].
>
> MAYA TIWARI, *AYURVEDA: A LIFE OF BALANCE*

Cow's milk represents Mother Earth herself in her aspect of spring or a new morning. She brings playfulness, hope, the planting of new ideas, innocence, and the feeling of awakening to the world anew and anticipating what the new day will bring. In her aspect of summer or high noon she brings the energy of productivity, getting the job done, and empowering the mind. In her aspect of fall, or twilight, she gifts the energy of bringing your energy inward, tying up loose ends, finishing projects, gathering your harvest or the fruits of your labor, and getting ready to rest. In her aspect of winter, or night, she brings the gifts of deep rest, sleep, hibernation, rejuvenation, dreaming, communing with deep mysteries, and shedding what is no longer useful from your previous cycle before you awaken again. We live these cyclic energies seasonally as well as daily as we are reminded when and how to be a child, an adult, and an elder and accept the responsibilities involved in each one of these cycles.

> For many people, cow's milk is the primary dairy they grew up with and still use. I invite you to feel into how the soma of this elixir has helped shape your life.

Goat Milk

Goat's milk helps you understand the forces of nature in their raw, unbridled, uncultivated forms of expression. This vibration is especially beneficial if you're afraid to camp, walk nature trails away from the city, swim in a lake, and so on. It's also beneficial for anyone who is working to release ingrained puritanical energies that have led to shame, or for anyone who suffers from panic attacks. According to archetypal psychologist James Hillman, panic attacks are often due to not being able to integrate one's own inherent wildness into the fabric of ordinary "decent" life. Opening to your inherent wildness allows you to draw succor from nature and be revitalized so as to develop the more vigorous aspects of yourself.

The goat is a strong theme in Greek mythology. Pan—primordial god of Earth, the wilds, and sexuality—is half man and half goat. His name simply means "all." In some myths he is known as Earth Father. Notably, he has never had a temple dedicated to him; instead, grottoes, clear lakes, meadows, woods, and caves are his places of worship. He offers the boon of helping us remember body wisdom so that we can get out of our heads and into our instinctual selves.

Sheep Milk

This form of dairy brings the energy to create the resources that makes your physical life comfortable—food, warmth, and shelter, the basis of all life and the safety and physical security needed to thrive. Sheep's milk encourages you to take stock of the general security and stability of your life. If any aspects such as finances, health, or home need to be shored up, this energy will provide the creative ingenuity and strength to do just that. From this place of security you will have the fertile ground needed to plant anything into your life you would like it to grow.

Sumerian history is rich with deities associated with sheep. Duttur is the Sumerian pastoral goddess of ewes, milk, and the arts of dairy. She is the mother of Dumuzi, an ancient Mesopotamian king with godlike powers who is associated with shepherds and a thriving flock. He was the primary consort of the fertility goddess Inanna, "Queen of Heaven and Earth." We find in the myth of Inanna the timeless story of the earth watching over us and taking care of us. Her promise is to make the world fertile and able to produce what sustains us and keeps us safe. The following is a beautiful snippet from a love song from Inanna to Dumuzi:

My husband, I will guard my sheepfold for you.
I will watch over your house of life, the storehouse,
The shining quivering place which delights Sumer—

The house which decides the fates of the land,
The house which gives the breath of life to the people.
I, the queen of the palace, will watch over your house.

FROM WOLKSTEIN AND KRAMER,
INANNA, QUEEN OF HEAVEN AND EARTH

Water Buffalo Milk

The energy of water buffalo milk, which is gaining popularity in the United States, is that of finding the true path. This is very simple: Stop. Listen. Learn. Act. This opens you to being contemplative and journeying inward, meditating on the subject you are exploring, and receiving the answer not only in your mind, but in every cell of your body. It then helps you act accordingly to achieve your desired outcome.

Water buffalos provide about 15 percent of the world's milk supply. Their milk has twice as much butterfat and 50 percent more protein than cow's milk. Most commercial milk and cheese production is from herds established in Italy more than a thousand years ago, from animals imported from Asia.

Yak Milk

This vibration is a doorway, a portal in essence, that allows you to travel to other dimensions of time and space, places that might not even exist in our third-dimensional reality. This energy emboldens you to take the first brave steps in this exploration, connects you deeply to universal energy, and provides the ability to ground yourself solidly and safely while you explore.

A rough translation of the Tibetan word for yak means "a wish-granting gem that gives you everything you want," due to how essential they are for the survival of the people of the Tibetan Plateau, similar to the role bison played for Native Americans. It is thought that ancient Qiang herdsmen domesticated yaks about ten thousand years ago. With their long, thick hair and three times the lung capacity and three times more red blood cells than a cow, yaks are able to thrive on the "roof of the world," about three miles above sea level, where they are able to flourish on a meager diet of grasses and sedges and to use their rough tongue to aid in licking lichens off rocks. Not only do yaks provide for every aspect of nomadic daily life, their milk has spiritual significance:

> Nomads begin each day by reciting prayers and offering milk to the unseen spirits of the land and sky. Their surplus butter is paid as tribute to the monasteries, where it is churned into butter tea [*po cha*] for the monks and is used to fuel the myriad lamps lit in offerings to the gods. Among nomads, a barrel of milk is presented by a suitor to his prospective bride. Only if she drinks of it can their lives be joined in marriage. Milk is also a key ingredient in preparing the essence-extract elixirs used in Tantric rites of rejuvenation.
>
> Ian Baker, *The Tibetan Art of Healing*

EGGS

Symbolically, the egg contains all that is possible. It is full of the promise of new life, expressing the rebirth of nature and the fruitfulness of the earth and all of creation. In many traditions the egg is a symbol for the whole universe—that is, the cosmic egg that in the egg yolk and egg white contains the balance of male and female, light and dark. The golden orb of the yolk represents the Divine Masculine, which is enfolded by the Divine Feminine, the egg white, in perfect balance.

Many of the species listed below have corresponding sections in the Fowl section, beginning on page 119. Energetically, the difference between eating the egg or the bird is that the energy imparted by the egg is still in embryonic stage, while the bird is the matured energy. An egg is fragile, holding the potential of new life and new opportunities. It must be coddled and looked after during its incubation period. After the incubation period is complete, it is time to come out of your shell and bring into the world what you have gestated.

Black-Headed Gull Egg

This egg teaches the skill of turning the most unlikely things to your advantage. Accordingly, this energy teaches you to be productive and creative while using limited resources to your full advantage. It stimulates ingenuity and the willingness to test your comfort zone. This energy brings to mind tennis star Arthur Ashe's statement, "Start where you are. Use what you have. Do what you can."

Chicken Egg

The chicken's egg brings the knowledge of how to run a household in all of its complexity, from raising children to managing the daily domestic affairs necessary for keeping things running smoothly. This even extends to a shared bed in the form of "sex magic," which teaches you how to invoke fertility (in any form required) and how to use this sacred energy.

Duck Egg

> The duck egg has many healthful qualities, including being high in omega-3 fatty acids, calcium, iron, magnesium, potassium, zinc, and vitamins A, B_{12}, E, D, and folate. Notably, unlike chicken eggs, duck eggs are alkaline, meaning they leave your body less acidic after eating them.

The duck's egg helps you navigate your emotions. If you feel out of place or lonely, this energy is powerful for opening a harmonic that leads you to situations and groups you have an infinity for. You can also tap into this vibration for any situation that requires working with your emotions, including intense depth work. One of my favorite aspects of working with this frequency is the fact that ducks are flat-out silly—nature's clowns. No matter what you're going through, duck-egg energy is always trying to help you find levity and joyful buoyancy.

Emu Egg

The emu's egg helps keep your family's energy clean unto itself and supports the understanding of what it means to be a clan. It is very helpful for the single parent who is raising a child alone or the primary caregiver with little support. It helps you cope with and find the energy to attend to the day-to-day tasks that are required, while working a full-time job and parenting.

Goose Egg

Geese bring the energy of abundance and are powerful for helping creative types birth ideas and figuring out how to monetize them. I know that is an uncomfortable topic for some people, but if you really incarnated to live a creative path and want to make a living from your ideas, goose eggs offer support. Their energy is fiercely protective, and they bring the sensation of security and being watched over while you walk your life path.

Guinea Hen Egg

The guinea hen's egg promotes respecting boundaries and understanding how to create sacred space.

Ostrich Egg

Eating the ostrich egg, the largest egg on Earth, gifts the energy of creating form out of chaos (the gap, void, formless primordial matter, pure potential) and holding that particular form until you're ready to allow it to dissolve and move into your next cycle. This egg also gifts the energy of wisdom, truth, integrity, and discernment.

The ostrich is sacred to the Egyptian goddess Ma'at. Her crown is an ostrich feather, and she used the feather to judge the souls of the dead, weighing the person's heart on the scales of justice against the ostrich feather. If your heart weighed more than the feather (a life poorly lived), you would be consumed by the demoness Ammut, known as "the Devourer" and the "Eater of Hearts." If your heart was light as a feather (a life lived well), you could enter into the afterlife. Ma'at is the goddess who set the order of the universe from chaos at the moment of creation and constantly prevented the universe from returning to chaos. Any time a deity has such a strong association with an earthly being, it is wise to explore this energy through a macrocosm/microcosm lens.

Quail Egg

Quail brings the energy of the fertility that comes through group dynamics, that each one contributes some aspect of care, food, warmth, shelter, and the safety and physical security needed to thrive.

FISH

Fish are aquatic craniate animals that lack limbs and can survive only in water. While the exact number is unknown, it is believed that about thirty-four thousand fish species exist around the globe. They have adapted to diverse aquatic environments, such as rocky shores, kelp forests, salty sea waters, and fresh rivers, streams, and ponds. Fish deepen our participation with the unconscious world. In many cultures fish are understood to help merge the principles of spirit and matter.

Alaska Pollock

This fish helps in overcoming sorrow, sadness, and discouragement.

Anchovy

Anchovy promotes finding a centered path or frame of mind so you don't become sidetracked by the myriad options available.

Arctic Char

Arctic char calms and quiets the emotions and mind, allowing you to experience deep stillness and silence.

Barramundi

The barramundi, or Asian sea bass, helps you realize that you contain both male and female energies within your psyche. This hermaphrodite reaches sexual maturity at around two years of age, at which time it is male. When it reaches approximately five years of age, it changes to female.

This fish brings the energy of completeness. It opens you to understanding the solar right side and the lunar left side that dwells within, and can also denote union or balance between the sexes, opening you to passion, sexuality, power, and regeneration. In essence, it is two becoming one.

Catfish

Catfish helps heal the pattern of not liking yourself so you play the rebel, using intellectual hostility, defiance, and criticism of others and life itself as a self-protection mechanism. Catfish rights this energy into a positive sense of self that in turn allows you to engage in life in a healthy, balanced way.

Cod

Cod helps resolve the issue of being overly competitive or dismissive, and encourages you to interact with others as equals so you can celebrate their achievements and interests.

Halibut

Halibut supports seeing lineage patterns, bringing awareness to those configurations that have their roots in many lifetimes (yours and your ancestors') and the knowledge of how to use these intersection points. It allows you to weave into your life the energy you would like to retain and cultivate, and to cut the Gordian knot of what you don't want.

Lingcod

Lingcod heals the energy of being afraid to be alone while simultaneously pushing away those who would take away your aloneness.

Mahi-Mahi

This fish stimulates positivity and focusing that energy out toward others, as well as becoming happy by giving.

Monkfish

Monkfish stimulates intuition and knowledge so you can maintain a clear head when in a challenging situation. It helps you find solutions and rise above conflict, teaching never to indulge in attempts to control, violate, or dominate.

Perch

Perch supports making decisions from your heart space while understanding the implications of those choices.

Rainbow Runner

This fish supports those who are exploring the edge of the unknown, and empowers authentic pioneers and adventurer types in both the physical and mental realms.

Rainbow Trout

This fish brings the ability to stay centered, even in the midst of life's wild and quickly flowing currents, granting opportunities to connect with your future. This may feel like subtle growth opportunities coupled with challenges, although trout will teach you how to manifest in all circumstances. It's not to your advantage to remain stuck in the same routines, fearing the significant changes flowing toward you. Meet whatever wonderful opportunity is coming your way with an open mind.

Red Snapper

Red snapper heals verbal aggression and hostility, and supports changing that behavior if you are the perpetrator, or healing the energetic fallout of being on the receiving end.

Rockfish

Rockfish promotes the ability to stay with a task or idea and not fantasize to the point where progress stops. It supports being idealistic and practical at the same time.

Salmon

Salmon asks you to be ready for adventure, open to the vast horizon of the unknown, and willing to take risks (in the subtle realms or the physical). In such situations it's common to feel lost, but you can feel more comfortable following the path that lies ahead of you and explore the amazing possibilities awaiting you. Never worry, your divine knowing will let you know when it's time to return home again. This could be literal or metaphorical, as in going back to the "home base" of your essence self, with one more layer of information for you to add to the creation of you.

Sand Dab

This fish offers tender support if you've experienced a deep hurt and assists you in reaching out for help rather than shutting down and moving deeper within. It encourages trusting a slow, gentle healing process.

Sardine

Sardine supports understanding group dynamics and the hive mentality, in which a group of people think and act as a community, sharing their knowledge, thoughts, and resources.

Sea Bass

Sea bass helps you appreciate the small miracles of each day and discovering life's treasures where you least expect them, restoring a sense of delight.

Shark

This is a fish for those who experience primal fear, terror, or grief that is paralyzing. Shark supports clearing deep trauma and bringing reorientation to your core, through all subtle levels down to the cellular, allowing profound changes to occur and a new level of freedom. This provides the ability to move forward in life.

Sheepshead

Sheepshead turns your perspective around to encourage the realization that the first and most important opinion is the one you have about yourself. From this lens come personal objectives for growth and expansion built on positivity, and self-assessment rather than outside recognition.

Sheepshead showed up in my life at a very pivotal point. One of my karmic lessons this go-round has been that in the past I tended to end up in relationships where my partner discouraged my ideas, from a flat-out "I won't support you in that venture, it's too out there, you should choose a more traditional, safer idea to cultivate" to "Your execution is lacking and you will fail, so don't even try." In hindsight I can now see how, being young and having that energy directed at me constantly, I could easily have become derailed and veered away from my passions. The universe, being unfailingly kind and supportive, opened a door for me, though I didn't know it at the time. Out of the blue I was invited to go on a fishing trip to La Paz, Mexico, and I happily accepted. Before that trip I had never heard of sheepshead and had definitely never tasted one (I believe in synchronicity over luck of the draw). I kept catching sheepshead almost exclusively (interestingly, not everyone on the boat did). A fun aspect of the place where we were staying was that you would bring your daily catch back and the kitchen would prepare it for your dinner. Needless to say, I ate a lot of sheepshead in a short amount of time! The sheepshead's diet consists mostly of shellfish and aquatic plants, so they tend to have a sweet, shellfish flavor and firm, moist flesh. The place where I stayed served it with a simple preparation of salt and lime (the energy of lime is to bring emotional clarity and shift you from being resentful, contracted, and apathetic). After I returned home, a subtle shift occurred for me, and I had the strength to reorganize my life. It took years for me to understand the energetic underpinnings that supported me not only in my decision-making process, but following through in the physical realm. In a significant way the sheepshead and lime combination opened the way for me by altering my subtle body, which literally led to a new way of being.

Sole

Sole supports overcoming shyness and being vibrant and outgoing.

Squid

Squid heals being demanding, excessively focusing on yourself and what you have or don't have, and using manipulation to achieve your wants.

Swordfish

Swordfish brings clarity and focus so you can harness your inner strength and sense of purpose, directing it toward goals. This is helpful if you tend to get derailed halfway through a thought process or project.

Tuna

Tuna asks you to move steadily along in life, uncover your secret resources, and create stability and financial security in your life. Doing this gives you the freedom to dream, fantasize, and be adventurous.

SHELLFISH

Shellfish is a broad term for various aquatic mollusks, crustaceans, and echinoderms that are used as food. An imprecisely defined culinary and fisheries term rather than a taxonomic one, the term refers to those aquatic invertebrates that have a shell or a shell-like exoskeleton, such as bivalves (clams, oysters), gastropods (snail, abalone), crabs, lobsters, shrimp, and sea urchins. Energetically, crabs are synonymous with the full moon and are linked to the changeable quality of the sea. In the clam we see the chaste beauty of the primordial shell, and it brings receptive, intimate, sensual, and creative energies—gingerly exposing itself and then not. In the oyster we find the ability to protect one's delicate self against irritants—and then turn the irritant into something exquisite. From the scallop shell we see *The Birth of Venus,* a painting by Sandro Botticelli, depicting Venus, the goddess of beauty, love, passion, and art being born.

Abalone

Abalone reminds you that you are responsible for what today will bring, and knowing this gives you a great responsibility in that you cannot blame your state of mind on anyone else; it all rests with you.

Abalone are marine snails, and their shells are often used in smudging rituals. Smudging is an indigenous tradition that involves burning herbs or resins—commonly, sage—to purify people or environments.

Clam (General)

Clams live in an intertidal zone, where land and sea meet, between high and low tide. They are under the water during high tide and uncovered on the tidal flats during low tide. They are adapted to huge daily changes in moisture, temperature, turbulence, and salinity. Energetically, clam imparts this oceanic memory of how to adapt to situations and thrive all the while. See specific clam varieties beginning on page 118.

Cockle

This heart-shaped bivalve can heal deep subconscious fears about your present situation that lead to an inability to move or think clearly. These fears might stem from acute loneliness, tight finances, or difficulty around the aging process. Cockle helps replace these feelings with a sense of calm that allows you to process information and move from a frozen state.

Conch

Conch seeds the spiritual understanding, desire, and energy to transform and work for global and community issues and not just for personal possessions and physical wants.

Crab

Crab teaches discernment of what is truly required in interpersonal processes versus what is expected. By taking spiritual responsibility instead of following personal egoic pressures, you are released from emotional and psychological entanglements and can cultivate detachment around these and other issues.

Crayfish/Crawdad

This shellfish helps heal the pain, deep hurt, and fear that occur due to betrayal (emotionally or physically), especially if the source is a group or person you trusted or loved. When such experiences imprint on the psyche/emotional body, it is often hard to open yourself again and allow yourself to be vulnerable. Crayfish helps heal these wounds and supports building relationships and reestablishing the emotional foundation you need to feel safe, trust, and share the soft intimate aspects of self.

Langostino

This is a crustacean that is neither a true lobster nor a prawn and is more closely related to the hermit crab.

Langostino releases the overwhelming need to control yourself and second-guess your every action, leading to a constricted form of expression that is not authentic but is instead produced by what the mind perceives you should be doing.

Lobster

Lobster heals the feeling that you are not inherently worthy of love, that you must always aggressively be doing something to earn love. It supports the sense of feeling safe in the knowledge that just being yourself is enough.

Lobster, Spiny/Rock

This crustacean is a powerful force for balancing the mental body, especially if you are easily distracted or disoriented, have difficulty concentrating, or experience cloudy thinking and tend toward compulsions, obsessions, and tantrums.

Mussel

The mussel helps heal deep anger, the kind that takes you almost to the tipping point of rage.

Oyster

Oyster opens you to oceanic ecstasy experienced as profound peace, tranquility, serenity, and radiant joy. You experience a blissful, tension-free state, a loss of ego boundaries, and an absolute sense of oneness with nature and the cosmic order. It is especially helpful if you desire a complete merging with another person.

Scallop

Scallop helps you understand the complex nature of romantic love, beauty, and eroticism, which are born from both the ethereal and the physical realms and connect you to powerful primal forces that propel you toward learning the lessons of love.

Sea Urchin

Sea urchin reminds you that a broken heart is an open heart. You must be willing to allow deep emotions to flow, and in doing so a gift of love is available from the other side. This is the bittersweet aspect of love. What seems lost will be regained many times over. A crucial aspect is allowing yourself the space to feel these emotions. Honor this time, and with faith and hope, a new revelation will gently come forward to heal your broken heart.

Shrimp

Shrimp restores and helps you retain sweetness and innocence during the wear and tear of normal daily life.

🦪 Clam Varieties

Butter Clam

The butter clam increases sensitivity, enabling you to understand what's involved in growing love and assisting you in taking down any barriers to letting love in.

Geoduck Clam

This variety energizes the first and second chakras, undoing energetic blockages in the lower back and spine, and healing reproductive ailments that have an energetic root, including infertility, frigidity, or lack of feeling, as well as acting as a balm on the subtle level for scars resulting from sexual trauma.

Razor Clam

Razor clam is helpful for the old soul who is world-weary, where it feels like you have seen and done everything life has to offer and are experiencing flat-out ennui. This mollusk allows you to tap into one more layer of living and find fresh experiences.

Venus Clam

Venus clam supports highly evolved and fragile souls, assisting with self-liberation, self-expression, and individuation, while retaining the refined and tender qualities of feminine beauty.

FOWL

The term *fowl* applies to domestic birds, such as chicken and turkey, as well as game, such as pheasant and duck. Birds are as at home in the water and air as they are on the earth. They bring the energy of being able to shift between states of being, forming a link between heaven (air) and earth, or the conscious (earth) and unconscious (water). Phrases such as "nesting" and "stretching your wings and learning to fly" have come to mean creating comfort and living your best life.

As discussed in the section on eggs, whether you ingest the egg or the bird, the same energy is imparted. In egg form this energy is still developing, and in fowl form it is mature.

Chicken

See the description for chicken egg on page 107.

Duck

See the description for duck egg on page 107.

Goose

See the description for goose egg on page 108.

Grouse

Grouse offers an invitation to look beyond your physical limitations to recognize your own immortal spirit. This energy supports opening a window onto the Divine and using this opportunity to find the abilities required to enhance your growth, then exercising those talents to the fullest. This vibration is also a call to engage in spiritual activities that help you transcend your mundane self.

Ostrich

See the description for ostrich egg on page 108.

Pheasant

Pheasant teaches that when it comes to relationships, it's not just giving that brings pleasure, but also receiving, and that together these two energies expand and join in a circle, and the exchange of energy grows exponentially, fueling the relationship.

Quail

See the description for quail egg on page 109.

Turkey

Turkey brings the energy of sharing with no strings attached, giving because it feels good to be in service to others without expectations. If you are stuck in the dynamic of giving with the hope of gaining, this energy will instill in your heart the sense that when something is done purely, with the right intention, it is a sacred action. Turkey also helps balance the energy of scarcity or greed.

OTHER PROTEINS

Protein is a foundational component of every cell in the body. It also helps form the energetic foundation in your life. Call upon protein to build structure and construct what you desire. All proteins strongly influence the root chakra.

Beef

Beef encourages the warmth and spirit of the home and celebrating the people you choose to have in your life. These connections remind us of who we are and bring us back to our roots, both culturally and personally, giving us a sense of continuity, of being part of something greater than ourselves.

Boar/Wild Pig

This animal offers an invitation to embrace the nature of the inner warrior and find the courage to face your fears and challenge them head-on. Boar stimulates the courage to face any situation that life brings your way and find a resolution.

Elk

Elk teaches the dynamic of when to engage in a conflict face-to-face because it's required to protect yourself, your loved ones, your ground, or your beliefs.

Goat

Goat connects to your raw, natural, wild-animal tendencies and reminds you that it is holy to accept these aspects of yourself, as they are gifts too. It allows you to embrace life in wild abandon and play.

Lamb

Lamb ushers in the energy of being renewed, allowing you, in the course of a single day, to feel reborn, supporting the sense of having a fresh start and imbuing the desire to use this opportunity to the fullest.

Pork/Domesticated Pig

Pig encourages you to actively work with your own intelligence, seeking ways of becoming smarter and expanding your personal knowledge. The knowledge associated with pork is especially helpful for creating material wealth and a comfortable physical life.

Rabbit

Rabbit offers an invitation to understand the moon (especially the full moon) on an archetypal level and all the gifts this brings. It teaches you how to embody abundance and fertility and how to bring these qualities into your life. An aspect of this is learning how to overcome timidity and fearfulness.

Seitan/Wheat Gluten

Seitan promotes enthusiasm in your endeavors, bringing beneficial energy to your current situation. It also brings awareness to any fine-tuning that may be required and encourages you to act on that knowledge with a smile.

Tempeh

This fermented soybean product offers spiritual connections as the root of group dynamics. These connections aid outward productivity, promoting receptivity to others' ideas and a willingness to share space and respect boundaries. This allows each person in the group to offer their unique gift, which ultimately amplifies the work of the whole.

Tofu/Bean Curd

Tofu promotes equanimity in all actions and has a calming, cooling, soothing effect on the mind and the emotions.

Venison

Deer brings the energy of tenderness in word, action, and deed, allowing you to be filled with kindness and radiate this much-needed energy out to all in need of it, so you can be philanthropic and perform works in behalf of humanity. It also brings sweetness to personal relationships that have grown brittle or harsh.

BEVERAGES

Few things are more enjoyable than a "cuppa." Tea and coffee bring the energy of enjoying group dynamics equally as much as spending time alone.

Coffee

Your morning cup of java, brewed from the seeds (not beans) of the coffee plant, can help you blend the creative power of thought, intuition, and divine inspiration within your heart for expression.

❦ *Tea Varieties*

After water, tea is the most consumed beverage in the world. The word *tea* can be a bit tricky, as to qualify as a true tea it must come from the *Camellia sinensis* plant, whereas teas made with herbs (for example, peppermint or chamomile) are technically tisanes. The following are true teas.

Black Tea

> The leaves of *C. sinensis* are crushed, curled, rolled, or torn and then left to oxidize before they're dried, giving black tea its strong, dark, intense flavor profile.

Black tea is for when your fiery yang aspects need to be reined in and directed with intent toward positive service, both inside and out.

Green Tea

> Green tea is prepared from fresh or slightly wilted leaves and then only lightly heated or steamed. This preparation stops the oxidation process and creates the lovely, subtle coloring and light, fresh, bright flavor profile of green tea.

This tea ushers in tenderness and love at a deep inner level, which aids you in opening to aspects of yourself that hold great sensitivity and insight into love, and then radiating this light out into the world through a luminous mind.

Oolong Tea

> Oolong is semioxidized and is most often produced as a whole-leaf tea. The level of oxidation impacts the flavor and color, so there is wide range of tastes and colors. The less oxidized the tea, the lighter in flavor and color; the more oxidized, the darker the color and bolder the flavor.

Oolong tea promotes a deep state of relaxation so you feel joyful, lighthearted, and peaceful.

Pu-erh Tea

Pu-erh tea is unique in that it undergoes a true fermentation process. Once the fresh leaves are picked, they are immediately placed in a large, heated wok to stop oxidation; then they're aged in a cold, humid climate. Traditionally, they would be aged in a cave for around three years, but now environmental controls allow this tea to be created at a much faster rate. The flavor is rich, dark, mellow, and mysterious; it tastes like history. It is most often sold as bricks or cakes. This is my favorite tea to order at a teahouse, as the presentation and energy are beautiful.

This brew connects you to the swirling energy of the universe and helps you remember that you're not alone in the world. You are unity and oneness, connected to every particle of light in every other being. We are in this together, and you have unimaginable support and opportunities if you just ask.

White Tea

White tea is a delicate, ethereal tea created from the buds (the hairs on the buds create a silvery white hue) and young leaves of the plant. They're steamed as soon as they're picked to stop oxidation, and then they are dried.

This tea brings the energy of whimsy and being fascinated at the small moments in life.

SELF-ASSESSMENT
Decoding Food Cravings

Think back to a time in your life when you had strong food cravings for a certain food, and reflect back on what you had going on at that time. Then look up the energetic signature of that food in this chapter and see how it relates. It is a fascinating practice to see how food truly has been your ally and supported your growth at a subtle level for your entire life.

During my childhood, when I could choose what my mom would make for dinner, I most often would request grilled chicken thighs in an apricot and mustard glaze. The energetic medicine I needed was the apricot and mustard, not the chicken. I was born into a very devout religious home, and the belief system I grew up with was not in harmony with my deep self. This caused a lot of confusion for me. I had a loving home and wonderful parents whom I loved dearly, but my soul was in agony due to the religious aspects of home life. What made it even more confusing was that I was the odd duck out, because everyone else in my family was fed at a soul level by our religious upbringing.

Mustard Seed: Mustard seed helps you connect to and address deep karmic issues that surface for resolution, and keeps your focus on what needs to be done in the moment to make changes.

Apricot: This downy, yellowish, sometimes rosy fruit brings balance and stabilizes mood swings and extreme emotional states. It promotes an exchange between the mental and subtle bodies, facilitates the reconciliation of internal conflicts and strong negative emotions that have been stored in the body, and empowers you to take responsibility for your life and make the changes necessary for health and well-being, thus fostering delight in life itself.

Narrative: Helps you connect to and address deep karmic issues and promotes an exchange between the mental and subtle bodies to facilitate the reconciliation of inner conflicts and strong negative emotions that have been stored in the body.

As you can see by the narrative, even at that tender age, before I could even fully process what was going on for me, the food I craved and ate was supporting me at an energetic level, so when I was finally old enough to process and work through that baggage I already had a head start.

When I was writing *Essential Oils in Spiritual Practice: Working with the Chakras, Divine Archetypes, and the Five Great Elements,* my primary nibbles as I wrote were corn nuts and dark chocolate (chocolate is not a taste I usually enjoy).

Corn: Corn, which comes in a multitude of varieties and colors, brings fertility and supports alignment with the earth's energies, opening you to the cornucopia that life offers and providing an earthy groundedness. A sacred plant of Native Americans, it ushers in abundance on all levels, especially the joy and pleasure associated with the feminine. Corn supports increased creativity and birthing the projects that result, and it is useful for fostering friendships and associations based on mutual support and growth by promoting the synergy needed to achieve goals larger than your own.

Cocoa "Bean": This plant teaches you how to live in joy; useful for those who tend to be bitter and have an over-somber sense of spirituality.

Narrative: Supports increased creativity and birthing the projects that follow, and for shifting an overly somber sense of spirituality.

Looking back, my deep self was keeping my "pen" in check and helping me to not write in a heavy, dry manner. The snack I craved the most as I wrote this book was popcorn, but not chocolate, as this subject matter is naturally light, and I didn't need the support of the cocoa bean, but I still needed an assist from corn.

This practice of recapitulation is so beneficial in getting to know yourself and seeing what you had going on at a subtle level during different times of your life.

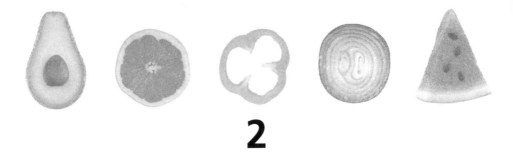

2

Divine Libation

Wine

You may have heard the word *totem* or *familiar* in relation to a specific animal and a person's special relationship with that being. Totems can also be plants, rocks or minerals, or other objects. Mine happens to be the grape, specifically in its alchemical role as wine.

I am not exactly sure why this plant chose me, but it chooses me as much as I choose it. I have always been magnetized to the myth, lore, and ritual concerning wine and I never pass up a chance to visit a winery or read up on the remarkable alchemical process of wine being made. Through this natural inclination and a numinous dream, I came to know that grape is one of my primary totems.

I am at the seashore, and beached on the sand is an immense albino blue whale. I know that she is trapped on the shore until the tide comes in to claim her and take her back to sea.

Suddenly, I find myself with two mythical sisters in a frail wooden house. The bottom of the house is submerged, and we are floating on the ocean. The windows have no glass panes. I look out of the window to see the Great Whale Woman swimming toward me with her two sisters, naked human women, riding on her back. I am terrified she will find me, and I hold my breath and close my eyes. All goes black.

Suddenly, one of my sisters opens her eyes and I know in a flash that the Great Whale Woman knows where we are. I am filled with such overwhelming fear. I open my eyes and see the Great Whale Woman, now with arms, pulling herself through the window. I wonder how she is going to fit into such a small fragile place and then realize that the only reason she can enter is because of the water on the floor. I am sure I will be destroyed, but I ask, "Before you kill me, may we have a drink?" Suddenly, all six of us—me, my two sisters, the Great Whale Woman, and her two sisters—are sitting in a circle. The Great Whale Woman has a chalice that she dips in the ocean water beneath us, and we pass it around and drink.

I knew in my dream that the ocean water we were drinking was symbolic for wine. The dream opened with the immense whale, representing divine information and knowledge, trapped on the shore, the conscious mind. Suddenly, I am submerged and the Great Whale Woman, representing the Divine Feminine in the ocean of archetypal knowledge, is coming for me. The Divine Feminine never had the intention of causing me harm, but the sensation of my smallness against the weight of her true divinity was overwhelming. The sacrament she offered me to get to know her was wine.

This dream helped me understand the function of wine for me. I love delving into the ocean of the collective unconscious and exploring archetypes, and I am primarily taught by dreams. This process of working with chthonic energies to uncover deep mystery is facilitated by wine for me.

I've spent much time getting to know this energy, and the following is an overview of some of the traits I think make the grape and its alchemy so special to me. Note that each plant has a different "voice," which may speak differently to each person; this is how the wine grape presents to me.

Sacred Plant: *Vitis vinifera*

Catalyst for: Cultivating the untrammeled self

Chakra correlation: Svadhishthana (pelvic bowl, second chakra); Manipura (solar plexus, third chakra)

Key vibrations: Vitis vinifera cultivates an expansive, sensuous, sensitive, spontaneous nature that delights in the beauty of everyday life. Be it the taste of the tart juice of the pomegranate, a perfectly balanced wine, the quickening that comes with your lover's embrace, or the simple beauty of a sunset, you see divinity in everything. *Vitis vinifera* teaches you to tolerate and even enjoy the outwardly "messy" as your edges come undone, and you begin to grow from deep, new, fecund places.

Key concepts: The energy of soulfulness. This is an expression of incredible depth, which provides softness toward the human experience. It's not the quest for perfection, but instead the practice of exploring what it means to be fully human within all of our individual variations; it is growing to love the seemingly disorderly and paradoxical aspects of human incarnation and staying in that process without shutting down, until the rich gift of experience can blossom.

Archetype: Dionysus, god of irrational wisdom, is the god of the grape, of wine-making and ritual ecstasy. Grapes have been used since antiquity to celebrate the Divine and to facilitate journeying to fantastical places where the conscious mind cannot navigate. The energy of the grape turning into wine "show[s] flowering in decay and fermentation, indestructibility in the midst of destruction."* This is a tale of death and rebirth, for whenever this plant is used as a sacrament or in ritual, it echoes the story of the grape turning into wine. Dionysus was celebrated yearly at Delphi, where he was worshipped as an adult god who died and spent time in the underworld and was born again as a newborn child: "In the inner sanctuary of Apollo's temple was the grave of Dionysus. For three winter months, Apollo handed over his temple to Dionysus while he went away far north, to the fabled land of Hyperboreans."†

*Cashford, *The Moon,* 32.
†Bolen, *Gods in Everyman,* 134.

This is a powerful vibration to work with, one that personifies paradox, as archetypally it expresses both the light (spirit) and the dark (soul). The two sides can help you reach mystical states and allow you to merge with the Divine in wild, joyful, orgasmic ecstasy, and in that moment you understand who you are in your most organic, feral state.

The grape in its fruit form brings the energy of the light: joy, levity, brightness, radiant health, love, and nurturing. This is the Dionysus who understands the secrets of nature, the friend of the nymphs and the champion of women whose souls are not honored. To understand this energy, let's get to know Dionysus a bit better. His mother was the mortal Semele and his father the god Zeus. His mother was consumed in divine fire after being tricked by Hera to have Zeus reveal his true form, a sight that no mortal can endure. Dionysus was then raised by the nature nymphs of Mt. Nysa. There he was tutored by Silenus, who was part man and part horse, and taught the secrets of nature and the making of wine. Dionysus, always the champion of women, descended into Hades to bring his mother back to life and take her to Olympus. He also rescued the abandoned Ariadne, a princess from Crete who was left on the island of Nexos by Theseus, where she would have killed herself out of despair if Dionysus had not saved and married her. In Greek mythology, Dionysus is the only god that rescues and restores, instead of dominating and raping, women. His primary worshippers were women from ancient Greece who communed with him in the wildest parts of the mountains.

Then an alchemical transition takes place, and the sweet sugars of the grape ferment and give birth to something mystical. This is the soulful side of the grape, or Dionysus in his grave. This darkness refers not to something negative, but to something deep, emotional, unfathomable, profound, fervent, heartfelt, sincere, and passionate, as well as meaningful, significant, eloquent, expressive, moving, stirring, sad, and mournful. The definition of *soul music* sums this up: "Broadly speaking, the soul comes from a [sic] gospel (the sacred) and blues (the profane). Blues was mainly a musical style that praised the fleshly desire whereas gospel was more oriented toward spiritual inspiration."[*] This is a vibration that allows you to intensely feel all of your emotions, not just the bright ones or the dark ones. It's an important part of soul health to be able to cry, to feel sincerely into injustice, sorrow, grief, and all other deep expressions. This is the death and rebirth cycle: darkness into light, light into darkness, as exemplified by the alchemical transformation of the grape into wine. In this way you can cycle through all the aspects of soul (dark) and spirit (light) with its natural rhythms.

What makes this vibration so fascinating to me is that there is no known female death-and-rebirth deity who has the grape as her vehicle. So the grape seems to act more in the role of *serving* the feminine as a kind of masculine consort of the Great Mother, or as feminist psychiatrist Jean Shinoda Bolen asserts: "Cybele or Rhea (both pre-Olympian great mother goddesses) . . . taught him [Dionysus] her mysteries and rites of initiation. Thus Dionysus was a *priest of the great goddess,* as well as a *god himself.*"[†] The grape has often called on women and men to step out of their ordinary lives to revel in nature, the Divine Feminine, and discover the ecstatic element within. In short, the grape serves as a priestess who initiates women and men so that they can experience the soul, i.e., the Great Goddess, who is embodied in each of us.

Incantation: Grape, I honor that you are the bringer of wildness and the most blessed deliverance. Your realm is the "life-giving and seminal moisture: the sap rising in a tree, the blood pounding in the veins, the liquid fire of the grape, all the mysterious and uncontrollable tides that flow and ebb in nature."[‡] I call on you to grant me your gifts and open me to life-giving nature so that I may find the passion that burns in my veins.

---

[*]Mark Nero, "Origins and Influence of Soul Music," liveabout.com website.
[†]Bolen, *Gods in Everyman,* 253.
[‡]Phillip Mayerson, quoted by Bolen, *Gods in Everyman,* 251–52.

♦♦♦

I encourage you to ask the plant, animal, or mineral kingdom to present to you your personal totem or familiar that you can work with to help you along your path in life.

EXERCISE
Meeting Your Food Familiar

The evolutionary process as a whole involves an interplay between creativity and habit. Without creativity, no new habits would come into being; all nature would follow repetitive patterns and behave as if it were governed by nonevolutionary laws. On the other hand, without the controlling influence of habit formation, creativity would lead to a chaotic process of change in which nothing ever stabilizes.

RUPERT SHELDRAKE,
THE REBIRTH OF NATURE

A dynamic way to find your food familiar is by exploring the space between the psyche and physical matter. Henri Corbin, a Sufi scholar, calls the middle space between the psyche and matter the mundus imaginalis; Carl Jung, a pioneer in depth psychology, named it the psychoid space; I call this area the liminal space. The word *liminal* is derived from the Latin word *limens,* meaning "threshold." When you're interacting with a liminal space, you're literally standing at a threshold between two realities. It is from this space that the visions, dreams, synchronicities, and magic that occur in everyday life become available. Gaining access to imaginal, creative experiences allows you to enter other realms of consciousness that are just as real as the world of the senses and the intellect. Doing this work gives voice to the soul and allows you to directly experience the creative impulse of the universe. This includes dream images, synchronistic events, mental pictures, and words and concepts arising in your mind, any of which are often coupled with a deep knowing that is often hard to express in words.

A notable aspect of working with liminal space is that you must knock on the door of the Divine asking for a relationship with your familiar. Your familiar, who serves as your guide, must answer this call. You cannot rush this process. After making your request, preferably in some sort of ritual way, cultivate inner spaciousness and wait in positive anticipation. Clues will come through your dreams (see chapter 3), through the crystallization of thoughts, and in the seemingly average events in your life that point the way (i.e., synchronicities).

Some of the ways to access your personal liminal space include dancing, drumming or rattling, automatic writing, fasting, floating in water or a sense-deprivation tank, or drawing or painting—basically any activity that takes you outside your rational mind. This is different from mind-training techniques such as using a mantra, chanting with intent, or reading. Here the idea is to engage in an activity that takes you out of the left-brain thought process.

This is how I did it:

1. First, I made a warm bath. Water is a power medium for me to access my liminal space.

2. I added fresh rose and marigold petals to access the energy centers I wanted to work with. Rose opens the heart and the crown chakra, providing access to divinely inspired information that resonates with what the heart truly needs or desires. Marigold stimulates the solar plexus chakra, which rules the conscious mind and integrating information for practical use.

3. I then settled into a quiet mind space and reverently asked for more of my food familiars to reveal themselves to me. Although wine/grape came to me in a dream and is very beneficial, I desired support to help me with more of my day-to-day affairs.

In the weeks that followed, two vegetable guides revealed themselves to me. Insights will often come to me while I'm doing the simplest of (nonmental) things, such as cooking, taking a bath, or gardening. Each person processes differently; there is no one way to receive information from your personal liminal space or a specific formula that will get you there. Simply follow the deep creative impulse that lies naturally within you. You are asking for a being to present itself, be it plant, animal, or mineral, who deeply supports your life path and personal growth. A familiar offers more than temporary support; it is a true guide and friend for life that is always there for you. Trust your knowing—when your familiar comes to you, joyfully welcome it into your life.

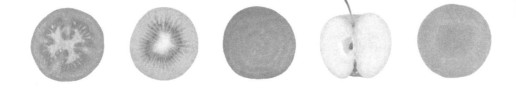

3
Building Your Archetypal Library

Working with Dreams

*C*ommunication *without words:* archetypes often show up as primordial symbols and aspects of nature in your dreams, coupled with sensations without any dialogue, leaving you to interpret what the Divine is trying to communicate to you. Which is why it's important to strive to learn the primordial language of dream symbolism if you would like to have a relationship with the ocean of wisdom that lies within you.

Working with dreams is one of the ways of decoding the energetic significance of the foods we eat. Working with pure energy is a right-brain, nonlinear activity that, as noted in the previous chapter, requires entering a liminal state. This is where dreams and their interpretations can be so helpful. Here is a dream that acquainted me with the energy of thyme.

> *I am at a gathering and a woman judge is presiding. She breaks up the crowd into groups and assigns each group a unique problem to solve. My dream sister and I, an older blond gentleman, and a few other people have to figure out how to dig a specific well (we have to come up with a creative solution as we can't just dig a hole into the earth) and then present our plan to the group. We come up with our idea and go to the*

front of the room to present our plan, but instead of speaking about our well blueprint, my sister and the older blond man start talking about their love. He goes on to explain to the group the difference between being spoken at and being spoken to. I become jealous and wonder why he didn't pick me and why he doesn't love me like that. The female judge tells him to stay on topic about our plan concerning the well, but he ignores her. Then, I am sitting right in front of him, face-to-face. He is still addressing my sister, but now I can feel what it would be like to be her. He then says, "We need you to come next Wednesday at 2:00," and he gives me a list of things to bring. He does all of this while looking down at this date book, just glancing at me and sort of waving his hand in my general direction. He then says that is me being spoken at. Then he says, "Candice, I would love it if you could come next Wednesday. It would make all the difference to me. It is important to me that you participate in this project, and besides, I love you." His eyes are very blue and unwavering and he maintains eye contact with me. I feel very connected to him and do not want the interaction to stop. He then tells me, that is being spoken to—and he hands me thyme.

As we learned in chapter 1, the energy signature for thyme is as follows:

....

Thyme: Thyme encourages warmth and receptivity, especially in the use of the spoken word. It teaches you how to use language to heal and creates the energy of inclusiveness and true caring. Thyme helps heal the compulsion to use cutting words, excessive sarcasm, and argumentativeness.

....

From my dream sequence, you can see how much I simplified the signature description. As you start to dream, fuller pictures and feelings will be given to you.

The collective unconscious is a timeless ocean of knowledge that encompasses everything in creation. It contains all this knowledge, with its countless stories, which create collective memories and impulses that dwell in each of us and in all of us. Jung defined the collective unconscious as follows:

> In addition to our immediate consciousness, which is of a thoroughly personal nature and which we believe to be the only empirical psyche (even if we tack on the personal unconscious as an appendix), there exists a second psychic system of a collective, universal, and impersonal nature which is identical in all individuals. This collective unconscious does not develop individually but is inherited. It consists of pre-existent forms, the archetypes, which can only become conscious secondarily and which give definite form to certain psychic contents.*

This explains why our frequencies are affected by other beings who also tap into this deep soul well, as each being is a unique emanation of the collective, or the one. This also makes it incredibly easy to share information on a subtle level.

The aspect of the collective unconscious that I would like to focus on involves communication from beings who show up in our dreams and help us understand the divine role of food in our life. Notably, once we assign meaning to something and understand what it represents, our deep self and the Divine will use it to communicate with us.

SHARING
Food Dream Takeaways

As you begin to study the energies put forward in this book and connect with them, they will show up in your dreams and start conversations with you. Often this will present as multiple images giving you direct instructions, teaching you or awakening in you an aspect that is ready to bloom. The following are some examples from my students:

---

*Jung, *Archetypes and the Collective Unconscious,* 57.

"I dreamed I was making conch fritters and passing them out to everyone who would take one."

....

Conch: Conch seeds the spiritual understanding, desire, and energy to transform and work for global and community issues and not just for personal possessions and physical wants.

....

Her takeaway: This alerted me to the fact that even though what I am working on is a job for me and helps support my physical needs, the aspect my deep self is excited about, my true desire, is that my project ultimately can support working with global and community issues.

◆

"I dreamed an oyster mushroom appeared and was hovering before me, and I watched it produce golden pollen. I plucked the mushroom from the air and knew I was supposed to bury it. I laid it in a hole that was already there and covered it with rich soil but realized I needed to fertilize it. So I walked down a row in a garden wondering what it needed, when I saw a cabbage plant. I knew it was correct. I picked four cabbage leaves and added them to the hole and started to place more soil on top but left it halfway empty."

....

Oyster Mushroom: Coming with the fall season and growing wild on trees, this mushroom asks you to look inside and feel into what you believe you truly deserve in life. Do you really believe you have the right to be happy? Loved? Fulfilled? To follow your dreams? If so, the oyster mushroom helps you nourish those seeds further. If at a core level you do not harbor these kinds of feelings, you will be aided by this spirit ally in planting the seeds that will eventually allow you to actualize what your deep self requires to thrive.

....

Cabbage: Both purple and green varieties help heal the sensation of loss of success or abundance and feelings that because you didn't succeed in the past you cannot succeed in the future. They support the need for individuality and a life-path direction informed by the soul.

Her takeaway: Since the hole was still halfway empty, I had the sensation that my deep self is just now ready to work with the soul questions that oyster mushroom poses about true fulfillment. It's a magical time, and I'm ready to allow myself to be filled to the brim with my true heart's desires and leave past failures and disappointments in the past.

◆

"I dreamed that I was walking in a field and found a calla lily and picked it. I continued to walk until I saw a beet. I dug it up and immediately I was filled with intense feelings of joy and fulfillment."

Beet: This intense vegetable opens the door to your inner realms, including past-life recall, and supports the conscious mind in exploring many aspects of the self previously unknown, restoring and integrating these aspects for use in daily life.

Her takeaway: Since I dreamed of picking a calla lily (its frequency is true love in a romantic relationship), I knew that the reason why it's been so hard for me to find my partner, my mate, is because I'm searching for a true love from my past life. I also know this will help me find him, and I feel sure I will. We will have the beautiful life my heart has yearned and ached for.

◆◆◆

In these dreams, the archetypal energy of the plant kingdom has clearly communicated with each dreamer, something they dearly desired but were not conscious of yet. Often archetypal dreams are answers to our silent prayers that we didn't even know we were sending out, but nonetheless they were received and answered. Once a dream is received by the dreamer, the Divine sets in motion what is required to respond to your prayers. You can support this process further by actually taking the nourishment that presents itself in your dream into your body. When I first started dreaming in this fashion, I often woke up to the refrain of "matter is the mediating factor." Anchoring the energy of your plant familiar or guide into your physical body is critically important; it helps magnetize to you situations and people that can assist in your journey and help rewire your subtle circuitry more efficiently. If for some reason you cannot find the particular nourishment that presented itself in your dream, or for whatever personal reasons you would rather not take it into your physical body, keep working with the energy that presents itself in its subtle form—you will get there! It will take just a little bit longer.

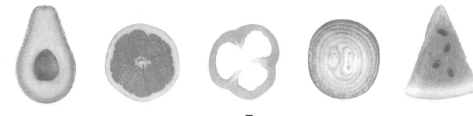

4

Eating the Rainbow

*Food Colors and
Chakra Correspondences*

The universe is the interplay between two fundamental principles: nature and supreme consciousness, or Source. They are two sides of the same coin. Supreme consciousness is the masculine principle that pervades all things; it is the sustainer. This is the ultimate, out of which mind and matter proceed. Nature is the feminine principle and forms this information; she is responsible for procreation, for birthing earthly existence. This is the basis of all creation, the power of evolution. This process is also referred to as Shiva-Shakti, yab-yum, yin-yang, Father Sky–Mother Earth—in essence, male and female energy combined, giving rise to experience.

The consciousness of a living being is set by the frequency of the matter that makes up the body. Our bodies allow us to engage in the play of nature, as no incarnation can be completely worldly or completely spiritual. No matter what level of light or spirituality you attain, you cannot transcend the human experience if you are embodied. Likewise, no matter how terrestrial you think you are, you are always filled with divinity. So the goal is to experience the balance of energy and matter working together to create a healthy whole, which allows curiosity, play, and exploration here on Earth.

An incredibly easy way to access these complementary energies is by working with the chakra system. Chakras are spinning wheels of energy, psychic centers that exist not on the physical plane, but rather in the spiritual dimension. The chakras set the frequencies that give rise to every aspect of the human experience.

The foods we eat have consciousness and provide an energetic blueprint that stabilizes and entrains matter and energy for us when consumed. The Vedic tradition teaches that we are all divine beings having a human experience. With this tenet in mind, we will focus on the seven main chakras, the energetic gateways that correspond to the spine. These allow us to process universal life-force frequencies. They allow us to experience and control the vast and wondrous energies available to us in our human experience.

What follows is an overview of the seven primary chakras and their functions. You will see that each chakra is assigned a color. An easy way to work with the chakras is simply to choose a food of the same color as the chakra you wish to stimulate—and then eat it! Sometimes it's the interior of the plant, not its exterior, that reveals its chakra correlation. For example, a kiwi fruit is brown on the outside, but its vibrant green interior alerts you to the fact that it vibrates to the fourth chakra, as that chakra's color correspondence is green.

Many fruits and vegetables come in multiple colors. In this case, if you find yourself with a craving or an aversion to a particular food, begin by reading the energetic signature to get the basic understanding of the plant's function, and then reference the chakra you feel drawn to based on its corresponding color for further information to round out your understanding. For example, bell peppers come in green, yellow, orange, red, purple, and white, and due to their respective colors each behaves in a slightly different manner.

There are many ways to work with a food's energy; let your intuition be your guide. You may choose to work with a food's energetic signature, provided in chapter 1, in combination with the energy of the specific chakra it correlates to. Or at times you may prefer to work with a food based solely on its color to access a specific chakra. While doing so can activate all the correlating chakra properties, all may not apply to you or your situation. Feel into and focus on what is relevant to you at this time.

CHAKRA ENERGIES

In the following chakra profiles I have provided a list of each chakra's energies—both the gifts and the shadow aspects, snapshots to understand the energies you're working with.* I include the name and location of each chakra and its elemental classification according to the Five Great Elements—earth, water, fire, air, wind, and ether/space.† I also include some representative foods that communicate these energies, although you will undoubtedly find more as you explore this territory.

Crown Chakra

Sanskrit name: Sahasrara

Number: Seventh

Location: Crown of the head

Element: Beyond the elements

Color: White

Representative foods: All white foods, including daikon radish, heart of palm, water chestnut, cauliflower, parsnip, lotus root, and jicama

This chakra holds the energy of detachment from illusion, an essential vibration in obtaining nonlocal consciousness and understanding the truth of one is all, and all is one.

---

*For a more detailed analysis of the chakras and their corresponding archetypes, sacred sounds, sacred geometry, and colors, see my book *Essential Oils in Spiritual Practice: Working with the Chakras, Divine Archetypes, and the Five Great Elements.*

†These five elements are the building blocks of reality and are known in Vedic literature as the *tattvas* (or *tattwas*).

Sahasrara translates as "thousand-petaled lotus." This is the most subtle chakra in the system, relating to pure consciousness, and it is from this chakra that all the other chakras emanate. When someone is able to raise their energy up to this point, they experience a state of enlightenment.

Third Eye Chakra

Sanskrit name: Ajna

Number: Sixth

Location: Center of the forehead (the third eye)

Element: All of the elements combined

Color: Purple

Representative foods: All purple foods, including eggplant, fig, purple potato, Wild Violet sweet corn, passion fruit, purple asparagus, and plum

This chakra holds the following gifts:
- Cosmic knowledge, control of the mind
- Seeing beyond duality; Shiva's eye (seeing past, present, and future)
- Sat-chit-ananda, "consciousness-being-bliss," embodying all the elements in their purest form; perfect concentration
- There is no observed or observer: "That I am; I am That"

Throat Chakra

Sanskrit name: Vishuddha

Number: Fifth

Location: Throat

Element: Ether

Colors: Blue and black

Representative foods: All black and blue foods, including black sesame seeds, forbidden rice, blueberry, borage flower, blackberry, black currant, and black grape

This chakra holds the following gifts:

- Truth, expression, sound, clarity, "giving voice to"
- True vocation, self-expression
- Clarity, wit, improvisation, spontaneity, active engagement with your inner muse
- Clairaudience, channeling, telepathy, working with subtle energies
- Understanding the power of words and how they shape and mold our reality

Shadow issues:

- Using words or sounds irresponsibly
- Not being an active listener, wordiness, and "speaking at" someone instead of real conversation
- Not able to discern truth; feeling muddled and confused
- Disengagement from your inner muse

Heart Chakra

Sanskrit name: Anahata

Number: Fourth

Location: Center of the breastbone

Element: Air

Colors: Green and pink

Representative foods: All green and pink foods, including kiwi fruit, avocado, lima bean, butter lettuce, pink grapefruit, dragon fruit, and guava

This chakra holds the following gifts:

- All love: unconditional, romantic, veneration of the Divine, parent/child, nature/pets, unattached, universal
- Fostering forgiveness, resolving conflicts
- Union with others and self, transforming the common into the Divine
- Experiencing the Divine in self and others
- Grace, surrender, compassion, loyalty

- Genuine concern for others and the desire to foster what is best for them

Shadow issues:

- Not accepting self, having only conditional love for self and others, rejecting the magic and beauty surrounding self
- Being controlling or jealous, demonstrating fear-based affection, using "affection" to manipulate, not allowing others to change or grow
- Feeling vulnerable or rejected, not allowing others in, not exposing "the real self," codependent relationships
- Being critical and hard to please, having an exaggerated view of people (whether positive or negative)

Solar Plexus Chakra

Sanskrit name: Manipura

Number: Third

Location: Solar plexus

Element: Fire

Color: Yellow

Representative foods: All yellow foods, including lemon, banana, yellow crookneck squash, yellow bell pepper, pineapple, and star fruit

This chakra holds the following gifts:

- Personal power, the intellect, opinion
- Logic, will, direction, leadership
- Action, authority, integrity, radiance
- Courage, self-worth, consciousness, and refinement

Shadow issues:

- Anger, volatility, rage, hatred
- Ego issues, abuse of power (e.g., domination, misguided force, using fear to control)
- Feeling superior, "my way or the highway"

- Perfectionism, rigidity, violence, and feeling weak
- Having no expression of personal choice

Sacral Chakra

Sanskrit name: Svadhishthana

Number: Second

Location: Sacrum/pelvic bowl

Element: Water

Color: Orange

Representative foods: All orange foods, including orange citrus, mango, papaya, peach, sweet potato, persimmon, and butternut squash

This chakra holds the following gifts:
- Sensuality, sexual intimacy, giving and receiving pleasure
- Creativity, unstructured expression
- Movement, things that wax and wane
- Healthy emotions and inner child
- "Hidden treasure" aspects of self, fluidity
- Working with dreams and the un/subconscious

Shadow issues:
- Wounded emotions, keeping secrets
- Fear of judgment, "getting in trouble," or "being found out"
- Repression of aspects of the self, inability to experience emotional or sexual intimacy, manipulation
- Nightmares or not being able to remember or interpret dreams

Root Chakra

Sanskrit name: Muladhara

Number: First

Location: Base of the spine/coccyx

Element: Earth

Color: Red/crimson

Representative foods: All red foods—including beet root, strawberry, Ruby Queen corn, cherry, pomegranate, watermelon, and cranberry— but especially root vegetables

This chakra holds the following gifts:
- Being grounded, earth connection
- Stability, security, a sense of belonging
- Raw sexuality, body pleasure
- Body knowledge, instinctual knowing
- Inner security and foundation of self
- Wise use of earth gifts (e.g., essential oils, crystals, metals/minerals, plant essences)

Shadow issues:
- Energetically anemic, feeling cut off and isolated
- Ambivalence toward life, poverty consciousness, substance abuse, or any type of drastic escapism
- Sex for any type of exchange or just to "feel"
- Not living in a sustainable way that supports the earth

THE DOSHAS AND THE SIX TASTES OF AYURVEDA

The ancient medical science of Ayurveda stems from the same Vedic sources as the chakra system. Ayurveda teaches that the three *doshas,* the three biological energies that define every person's makeup, are derived from the five elements, which are found throughout the human body and mind. These comprise our psycho-physical constitution.

Although every one of us contains within us all five elements— which in turn produce the lower five chakras, which in turn produce the doshas—the average person generally has two dosha types that predominate. You might, for instance, be a kapha-vata type or a pitta-vata type. Very rarely is a person truly tridoshic or a single dosha type, although due to seasons and lifestyle factors you can shift in and out of a variety of dominant combinations for a time. You may also achieve a state of equilibrium when all three doshas are in balance.

- Ether produces the fifth chakra, which produces the vata dosha.
- Air produces the fourth chakra, which produces the vata dosha.
- Fire produces the third chakra, which produces the pitta dosha.
- Water produces the second chakra, which produces the kapha and pitta doshas.
- Earth produces the first chakra, which produces the kapha dosha.

The elemental energies, representing the most primal aspects of self, give rise to the more refined chakra energies within the self, which in turn manifest as the doshas and their associated characteristics.

Vata body type is produced by the fourth and fifth chakras and is pacified by warm, oily, heavy foods and sweet, sour, salty tastes.

Pitta body type is produced by the second and third chakras and is pacified by cooling foods that are drying, with prominently sweet, bitter, and astringent tastes.

Kapha body type is produced by the first and second chakras and is pacified by light, dry, warm foods and pungent, bitter, and astringent tastes.

As a quick snapshot, the six tastes in Ayurveda are as follows:

1. **Sweet** is found in proteins, carbohydrates, and fats and builds tissues. Found in grains, breads, dairy, starchy vegetables, fruits, nuts, oils, sugar, honey, and animal products.
2. **Sour** is found in organic acids and promotes appetite and digestion. Found in citrus fruits, sour fruits, tomatoes, yogurt, cheese, pickles, vinegar, and alcohol.
3. **Salty** is found in mineral and ocean salts, is mildly laxative

and sedating, and promotes digestion. Found in salt, seafood, sauces, and meat.

4. **Pungent** is found in the essential oils of plants and stimulates digestion, clears congestion, and is detoxifying. Found in hot peppers, ginger, radishes, mustard, and all herbs and spices.

5. **Bitter** is found in alkaloids and glycosides and is anti-inflammatory and detoxifying. Found in green and yellow vegetables.

6. **Astringent** is found in tannins and fiber and is constricting and compacting. Found in beans and legumes (especially lentils), pomegranates, cranberries, tea, and dark leafy greens.

Not included on the list but fascinating is *umami*, a flavor sensation best described as rich and meaty, or "mouthfulness" and "heartiness." It is almost as much a feeling as it is a taste. It is said to derive from the amino acid glutamate, a key building block of proteins that enhances flavors already in the mouth, providing a sensation of richness. Braised, aged, or slow-cooked foods supposedly contain greater natural levels of this rich savoriness, as do foods like garlic, onions, mushrooms, scallops, tomatoes, and, famously so, parmesan cheese.

I've included this brief foray into Ayurveda to give you just a glimpse into some of the other fascinating connections that you might draw upon in your journey of self-discovery working with the energies of food. We'll now move on to a practice to help you connect to the energies of nature and select foods to enhance your own vital energy flow.

USING RITUAL TO "HEAR" THE LANGUAGE OF NATURE

To understand the language of nature and communicate with her, it's best to have an open heart. You must be willing to use your inner senses and intuitive feelings. This is the domain of ritual, where we can expand our consciousness in order to "hear" the tender teachings of our fellow life forms: "Ritual allows the right brain hemisphere to become dominate. This is the alogical [being outside the bounds of that to which logic can apply], holistic, intuitive, imaginative, feeling side of our cerebral cortex. The result is that we are in a transcendent state favoring new appraisals and fresh evaluation of our current circumstances."*

The following exercise is a guided meditation—a form of ritual—that will help you access your liminal space, allowing you to clearly hear your food guides. After selecting your food guides, you will use your body to see what chakra energies want to engage with you. These silent forms of communication will help you understand what your deep self wishes to say to you.

EXERCISE
. . . .
Food Selection for Vital Energy Flow

1. Choose an environment you find sacred. This could be lying on your back under the shade of a tree, submerging your bare feet in a stream, sitting at your kitchen table with a cup of tea with the sunlight streaming in, relaxing in a scented bath, or snuggling up in front of a fire. The key here is to not manufacture an environment, but instead to allow yourself to be drawn to whichever environment feels best to you in the moment. Once you find your place, allow yourself to settle and feel at peace.

2. Close your eyes and place your right hand on your heart and your left hand on your stomach, breathing effortlessly until you feel ready to proceed. Then ask the question, *What is hidden from my view that my deep self desires or that I need help with?* This will allow your deep self and nature to communicate with you. Please, if you have a genuine need for help or inquiry, frame your question as clearly as possible and ask now. Remember, your chakras and the food you eat influence all aspects of your life, so asking this heartfelt question provides an opportunity for your deep self to bypass your mind and lead you to the vital energies you need to work with.

---

*Mumford, *Magical Tattwas*, 55.

3. Using your mind's eye, transport yourself to a lush garden that has every fruit and vegetable imaginable. Allow yourself to stroll lazily around the garden, touching the leaves, taking in the scents, feeling the richness of the soil under your feet and the sun warming your face. No rush. Explore in this way until you find the fruit(s) and/or vegetable(s) that you are magnetized to. Pluck them and place them in your imaginary basket for later use. Also, check to see if you feel put off by any plant, and if so, add that to your basket. Remember, this is a spiritual exercise, so it doesn't have to be logical and based on your actual preferences. Feel into the spirit of each plant as you select, as all things are in each thing. You are in the plant, and the plant is in you, so this energy is excited to communicate with you.

4. If you feel satisfied you've completed your selections, you can stop looking in the garden; if not, allow your mind to continue to wander. Do you feel like fishing? Do you feel like clamming? Do you feel like wildcrafting? Do you feel like hunting? Do you want to visit your favorite ranch or farm? If any of these thoughts energize you, allow yourself to similarly explore the environment in which those things are found and add whatever you are attracted to or put off by to your basket. When you've completed all your selections, in your mind's eye, put your basket down.

5. Take a few deep breaths and ask your energetic body to reveal to you what chakra(s) would like to work with you. Then cup your actual physical hands and place them over your eyes. Wait for a color or colors to arise in your mind's eye or behind your eyelids. If it doesn't come readily, you can press lightly on your eyelids with the tips of your fingers for a few seconds and then release. Usually I am presented with a black background and color(s) that swirl and move. Make a mental note of whichever color(s) presents itself.

6. Thank nature softly for sharing her wisdom with you, and when you feel ready, open your eyes.

7. Write down which energies came to you, including both foods and colors. The act of writing helps your unconscious mind assimilate the underlying meanings. Look up the energetic signatures of everything that presented themselves to you in the visualization. Deeply feel into the energy of each item

and see what messages come with each. The messages will make themselves known—the colors will reveal which chakras would like to be worked with, and the foods will give you direction as to how to work with those energies. Nature delights in divine play like this, so now you can come up with some menus that incorporate the foods that support your question.

5

Deconstructing Recipes

Exploring the Narrative of
Some Common Food Groupings

Exploring the narrative of food groupings and the gifts they offer is a fascinating practice. I have found it to be very comforting and supportive in tending the garden of the self, and even more so in caring for those I love and want to nurture. Having a concrete way to support someone without being wordy or intrusive is powerful. Cooking for others can also be a way to reach out and support individuals and organizations you may not know as intimately but would like to help.

An example of how this works in my daily life: As I write this, earlier today I was beating myself up (even though I know better!) because I forgot a telephone appointment due to getting lost in my creative process. Halfway through my internal chiding, the image of a cremini mushroom came to mind, accompanied by a craving for cremini mushrooms dipped in creamy horseradish sauce. That calmed me and stopped my mind immediately, as I'm familiar with the energy of this mushroom:

....

Cremini: A cross between a white button and a portobello, cremini heals the energy of attacking the negative in yourself so that you can see and feel yourself in a gentler light, cultivating compassion for having those less-than-desirable traits and allowing kindness and softness to be a healing balm to relentless self-criticism.

....

And horseradish's energy:

....

Horseradish: Horseradish ushers in the energy of the Divine Masculine, being a protector and champion for others and yourself.

....

This gave me pause. I could then gather myself, and from a neutral, nonpanicky place I called my friend to explain what had happened and apologize for missing our scheduled call. Even though I was alerted at an energetic level as to what was going on, I find it's best whenever possible to follow up by actually eating the food(s) that have presented themselves. So that night for dinner I made a sauté using

cremini mushrooms, which heal the energy of attacking the negative in yourself;

royal trumpet mushrooms, which regulate your work cycle and give you a better understanding of time management;

onion, which helps you target specific aspects of yourself you want to work with;

parsley, for forgiveness and resolution of conflict;

rosemary, for remembrance;

and a drizzle of **horseradish** sauce, which ushers in the Divine Masculine as a protector and champion.

In this way I was able to forgive myself for mismanaging my time and understand how I got myself into that situation, as well as work on positive solutions so it wouldn't happen in the future.

The food we eat does and will rise to the occasion to support us in the day-to-day work of fine-tuning our behavior and thoughts. Of course, we can also use this method to work with and address aspects of self that require deeper healing and prolonged attention. I have found in my work with clients that the more you engage in this practice, the more your palate will expand. This allows you to go beyond traditional groupings and cook to truly nourish your deep self.

In this chapter we'll explore the synergy of food groupings and the narrative they create, using some common recipes. When you "read" the energy of a recipe, not every ingredient needs to be factored in to understand how it will behave as a whole. If a food is consumed that is not relevant to you on a subtle level, it will register as energetically neutral and will only nourish the physical body. So there's no need to be concerned about fine-tuning your recipes to the *nth* degree, so that it's no longer enjoyable to cook.

The following examples come from members of my study group, friends, and family members. Without telling them why we were doing so, I asked each person to select a recipe based on a recent craving and circle the items that jumped out at them. I then provided them with the energetic signatures listed in chapter 1 of this book and asked them to look up the items they circled and write down the aspects of the food signatures they related to. The next step was to look at the overall energies of each recipe and share the energetic narrative that comes with it, and then think about how that narrative was relevant to the person's life and how they could apply this energy. I have used a plus sign (+) to denote the foods circled by the person.

🌿 Shrimp Cocktail

Ketchup (tomato) +
Horseradish +
Worcestershire sauce (anchovies, molasses,
    tamarind) +
Lemon
Tabasco sauce (tabasco pepper) +
Shrimp +

Tomato = Dance of relationship. **Horseradish** = Divine Masculine. **Tamarind** = The ability to act from a clear sense of what you want. **Tabasco pepper** = Energizes and balances the first chakra and supports your ability to ground spiritual energy and higher love into the physical body. **Shrimp** = Sweetness.

Narrative: At this time in my life I am ready for an evolved love relationship, and I am ready to put in the work to cultivate and maintain this kind of relationship.

🌿 Lobster Lettuce Wraps

Butter lettuce +
Lobster +
Lemon juice +
Tarragon +
Mayonnaise

Butter lettuce = Restoring the "milk of human kindness" to your heart when you feel completely depleted. **Lobster** = Not having to do anything special to be loved, being loved for being myself. **Lemon** = The ability to laugh again. **Tarragon** = The return of my sense of humor and feeling uplifted.

Narrative: I want to be happy and have my soul filled up and soothed, so I can feel contentment from within. Eventually I would like to be able to share my joy and love with someone who can really see me and appreciate me for who I truly am.

❦ Caprese Salad

Tomato, Green Zebra +
Mozzarella cheese +
Basil +
Extra-virgin olive oil
Salt

Green Zebra tomato = *Releasing the restrictions and limits imposed on me.*
Mozzarella cheese = *Tapping into my family's energy.* **Basil** = *Unconditional, unrestricted love.*

Narrative: As much as I love my family, I would like more autonomy and freedom to be myself.

❦ Baked Portobello Mushrooms and Spinach

Portobello mushroom +
Olive oil
Onion
Spinach +
Garlic +
White wine
Parmesan cheese +

Portobello mushroom = *Truly understanding what I need to thrive and owning that.* **Spinach** = *For nurturing.* **Garlic** = *Letting my light shine.*
Parmesan cheese = *The comfort of belonging.*

Narrative: I have recently moved and am homesick. I would like to make more friends, feel settled in, and build a community I feel at home in.

🌿 Lamb Shank

Lamb shank +
Butter
Onion
Carrot +
Garlic +
Flour
Tomato paste
Bouquet garni (celery, thyme +, bay leaves, parsley +,
    cilantro, tarragon)
Red wine +
Beef broth

Lamb shank = Being renewed and allowing myself to be reborn and turn a new page in the course of a single day. **Carrot** = Seeing what is a healthy concern. **Garlic** = Protection from bad energy. **Thyme** = Speaking kind words. **Parsley** = I would like to be forgiven. **Red wine** = Rebirth, another chance.

Narrative: I've been really careless and mean with my words to my boyfriend, and I'm afraid I've hurt his feelings to the point that he's through with me. I would like another chance to make things right, and this time speak with kindness.

🌿 Pears Poached in Port with Zabaglione

Pear +
Lemon +
Sugar, white
Port wine
Red wine
Cinnamon
Cloves +
Egg yolks
Marsala wine +
Whipping cream, heavy
Hazelnuts +

Pear = Using spiritual guidance to explore life. **Lemon** = Goals and desires are reached by gathering all of my energy, then directing all of this centered energy and intellectual focus to my intended goal. **Cloves** = Deepening the creative impulse. **Marsala wine** = New perspective, thinking outside the box. **Hazelnut** = Fosters the development of skills, supports all form of study and the ability to retain useful information.

Narrative: I love this! I just started taking watercolor classes, and this recipe will help me learn the techniques being taught and allow me to tap into and explore my creativity.

🌿 Arborio-Crusted Oysters

Oysters +
Flour
Arborio rice +
Sesame oil
Garlic +
Cremini mushrooms
Clam juice
Vegetable stock
Lemongrass +
Ginger
Rice wine vinegar
Soy sauce
Roma tomatoes
Green onions +
Cilantro +
Spinach

Oyster = Opens me to oceanic ecstasy, experienced as profound peace, tranquility, serenity, and radiant joy. **Rice** = Encourages serenity and harmony, realigns and strengthens my energy flow and brings simplicity. **Garlic** = Inner light. **Lemongrass** = Heals my lack of self-control and volatile expressions of self. **Green onion** = Brings me back in touch with loved ones, promoting sensitivity; allows me to be in the here and now; patiently allowing time and space for closeness and the little joys of life together. **Cilantro** = Helps me balance my poor internal anchoring and being overly swayed by environmental factors.

Narrative: I've been very triggered by the sensation of being ignored and not a priority with my partner, and I have been acting out to get his attention. I think this recipe will help me calm down, be patient with him, and explore better ways to get my needs met.

🌿 *Succotash*

Lima beans +
Butter +
Onion
Red bell pepper
Corn +
Paprika +
Garlic
Thyme +
Black pepper

Lima bean = *Promotes living in a state of wonder, curiosity, and flow.*
Butter = *Sweetness of life.* **Corn** = *Taking in all that life offers.* **Paprika** = *Passion, enthusiasm, and warmth.* **Thyme** = *Warmth and receptivity.*

Narrative: I'm ready to open up and take in all of life and see where that takes me without being in my head so much. I would like to learn how to live in the energy of divine direction and explore that.

🌿 Chicken Cassoulet with Butter Beans

Onion +
Pancetta (pork) +
Whole chicken +
Italian parsley +
Thyme
Garlic
Lemon
Bay leaf +
Butter beans +
Cherry tomatoes +
Chicken stock
Olive oil
Salt and pepper
Potatoes

Onion = Exploring inside. **Pancetta/pork** = Helpful for creating a comfortable physical life. **Chicken** = Keeping a household running smoothly. **Parsley** = Resolving conflicts. **Bay leaf** = Deeply energizing on many levels, clearing blocked or stagnant energies and renewing vitality. **Butter bean** = Brings the desire to share with others what you deeply love (whatever it may be) with warmth and enthusiasm. **Cherry tomato** = Love.

Narrative: Much of what makes a house a home isn't present where I live now. It feels cold and sterile. Our children have grown up and left, and my husband and I have grown apart. I dearly want to bring the energy of warmth, joy, and love back into our home.

EXERCISE
......
Reading a Recipe's Energies

1. Choose a recipe you've already been thinking about making, and list the ingredients on a piece of paper.

2. Close your eyes, take a few deep breaths, and consciously connect your energy to the energies of the ingredients you listed.

3. After you feel connected, open your eyes and feel into each item listed. Circle any that feel particularly energized to you.

4. For each ingredient you circled, look up the corresponding energy signature in chapter 1 and write down any aspects that stand out for you.

5. Review what you transcribed, taking all of the energies into account. Read them as a whole to find the narrative.

6. Write down the narrative you discovered and contemplate how this energy would support you currently.

6

Recipes

*Creating the Fabric of Your
Being with Vibrational Nutrition*

When we cook for our family and friends, most often it is as a show of affection, to celebrate, to bring comfort, to aid in mourning, or to create space for quality time and really being together. Food is a cornerstone of human interaction in so many ways—it's poetry, really. How often, when words or actions were not enough, did you invite someone to break bread and express a deep feeling?

This chapter is designed to help you connect more consciously to why recipes make us feel certain ways so that you can cook from the heart and not just from a taste perspective (although that will be a factor, of course). In this way you'll be able to create meals that express your deepest sentiments. The recipe collection here is an expression of experiences from the kitchens of the cooks I love. Each recipe tells a story. I have focused on some out-of-the-ordinary dishes that perhaps might be hard to find a recipe for. Note that any recipe can be made vegan or vegetarian by simply eliminating or substituting another ingredient for protein or dairy. I include measurements, but these should be taken with a "grain of salt," so to speak—that is, as loose guidelines.

Cooking is a creative act and I feel that it needs room for much flexibility, which also allows us to cater to those we are cooking for. I have not provided the number of "servings" for these recipes, as we all know this can vary so greatly by individual and by family. Nor have I attempted to tell you how long it should take you to prepare the recipes. Making a dish for the sheer joy of it, you will stretch out the act, perhaps listening to Nina Simone while sipping a nice red. When you are in a rush and have to tend to your day, you will chop quickly and get it taken care of. This act of joyfully adjusting to your environment and feeling what is needed at any certain time is half the fun! So I have only provided loose guidelines. My hope is that you will feel into your environment and celebrate each moment as it is.

Allow your palate and intuition to lead the way, and be not only willing, but eager to substitute different vegetables, proteins, spices, and so on, to fine-tune the recipes to truly suit your individual tastes and needs and those of your family and friends.

I have included a general energetic outline and narrative of each recipe, and you can consult chapter 1 if you want a more in-depth reading of the energetic signature of each ingredient. Also keep in mind that each food item may have multiple layers of information, so tune in to the aspect that applies to you in that moment or is specific to a certain recipe.

Bon appétit!

MATTERS OF THE HEART

🌿 *Apples of Love Soup (Tomato Soup)*

10 sun-dried tomatoes
White wine
1 medium purple onion
2 tablespoons avocado oil
2 small Yukon Gold potatoes, peeled and diced
1 teaspoon dried basil
1 teaspoon dried thyme
4 large cloves garlic, crushed
28-ounce can diced tomatoes
1 tablespoon sea salt
½ teaspoon ground black pepper
1½ teaspoons brown sugar
2 cups vegetable stock
Fresh basil, for garnish

Coarsely chop the sun-dried tomatoes; in a small saucepan, cover eight of them with white wine and simmer for 3 to 4 minutes, until soft. Reserve the liquid. Coarsely chop the onion, add to a large soup pot with the avocado oil, and sauté for 3 minutes. Add the potatoes and herbs and continue cooking for 4 minutes. Add the garlic, softened tomatoes, and reserved liquid, and sauté until the garlic is fragrant. Add the diced tomatoes, salt, pepper, and brown sugar and cook for 4 to 5 minutes, stirring often. Finally, add the vegetable stock and simmer for 15 to 20 minutes. Either use an immersion blender and blend right in the pot until smooth, or blend in batches in an upright blender. Adjust the seasonings to taste. Garnish with the remaining dried tomatoes, cut into thin strips, and some fresh basil.

Narrative: This soup is perfect for any matters of the heart. Tomato, first and foremost, teaches togetherness in many forms. Be it a loving family, a robust community, the dance of a relationship, a passion, or even courtship, this fruity vegetable is all about the heart. A part of this dynamic is its ability to help you be open to differences and new circumstances and joyfully embrace them.

🌿 Shaved Asparagus with Garlic Scapes on Naan

About ½ pound asparagus
Olive oil
Salt
Ground black pepper
Garlic powder
6 garlic scapes
Good-quality mozzarella cheese
Naan bread
1 small bunch of tender thyme in bloom, chopped
5 chives in bloom, chopped
Parmesan cheese

Wash the asparagus; do not snap off the tough ends yet, as you'll use them as a handle. Using a vegetable peeler, hold the tough end and peel the asparagus the long way into strips. I can usually get 3 or 4 strips per stalk, depending on the width. They do not need to be uniform in shape or size. Now cut off the tough ends. Place the asparagus strips in a large mixing bowl and toss with olive oil until fully coated. Salt and pepper liberally and add about ½ teaspoon (or more) of garlic powder. Mix to make sure each strand is evenly coated.

Wash the garlic scapes and trim the ends. Place in a large mixing bowl, toss with olive oil, and add salt and pepper to taste.

Cut the mozzarella in thin slices. Depending on how large the naan is, cut enough slices that you will be able to cover the top with no large gaps.

Using a pastry brush, spread olive oil evenly over the naan, lay the mozzarella cheese evenly on top, and then arrange the asparagus, garlic scapes, tender thyme, and chives over the cheese. Grate a nice sprinkling of parmesan cheese on top of everything. Bake at 425°F for 15 to 25 minutes.

Narrative: This dish heals myopic states that hinder and harm the relationships in your life (they feel it, even if you keep your opinions to yourself) by opening your eyes to see the vastness of people you interact with so you can appreciate and see them for who they really are. In so doing, your energy will change in your relationships with others, and a whole new level of intimacy will bloom.

You might serve this dish when you have the jarring realization that you've been projecting on someone and need support in clearing that energy so you can see with clear eyes.

🌿 Lingcod and Vegetables Baked in Parchment

> 2 filets lingcod
> 1 lemon
> Salt and ground black pepper
> Olive oil
> 2 large sprigs rosemary
> Tomatoes
> Banana peppers
> Broccoli
> Green beans

Rinse and pat dry the two fish filets, place them on a sheet of parchment paper three times their size, and place in a shallow glass pan. Squeeze lemon juice on both sides and season with salt and pepper to taste. Drizzle olive oil over both filets, and place a large sprig of rosemary roughly the size of each filet on top.

Layer the vegetables on top in this order: 1) tomatoes; 2) banana peppers; 3) broccoli; 4) green beans. The amount of vegetables you use and the shape you cut them in is entirely up to you.

Drizzle a bit more olive oil on top of the vegetables, squeeze lemon juice liberally on top, and finish with salt and pepper.

Wrap snugly in the parchment paper and bake at 400°F for 15 minutes. Remove and open the package and spoon the juices over the entire mixture. Using the edges of the parchment paper, create a wall around the fish and vegetables, leaving the center open and the mixture exposed. Put back in the oven for 15 more minutes.

Narrative: This dish promotes a radiant, open heart that is free from the heavier aspects of the emotions, helping you achieve a balanced togetherness, love given freely and received, and emotional openness. You might serve this dish after a quarrel, if you would like to coax someone out of their shell, or if projection is occurring (e.g., anger, jealousy, etc.). It is also perfect for bringing up any topic that you want a receptive audience for.

🌿 Robust Venison Chili with Corn and Chickpeas

Venison is a very lean meat that benefits from fat being added. We get that from the roux and the chickpeas, which have a naturally rich, buttery taste and texture that enhance the natural qualities of venison. The corn adds a bit of sweetness that brings out the grassy notes in this chili.

1 ½ pounds venison
Olive oil
Salt and ground black pepper
½ teaspoon garlic powder
1 white onion, chopped
3 low-water tomatoes (such as Roma), diced
3 cloves garlic, peeled and smashed
2 serrano peppers, roasted and chopped
1 jalapeño pepper, roasted and chopped
2 sprigs fresh oregano
3 teaspoons chili powder
½ teaspoon paprika
¼ teaspoon dried mustard
1 tablespoon soy sauce or Bragg's Liquid Aminos
1 cup salsa
3 tablespoons flour
6 cups vegetable or beef broth
½ cup frozen or fresh corn
2 cups cooked chickpeas

In a large pot, brown the venison in olive oil, liberally sprinkling it with salt, pepper, and garlic powder on both sides. Then remove the venison from the pot. Keep the brown bits and juices.

Add more olive oil as needed to the pot throughout this process: Sauté the onion until soft, then add the tomatoes, garlic, peppers, herbs, spices, and soy sauce and cook, stirring often, for 3 to 5 minutes. Then add the salsa and continue cooking for 3 to 5 minutes, stirring frequently. Finally, add the flour gradually, stirring constantly until a rich paste is formed. Add the broth a little at a time, stirring continually until the paste is absorbed and smooth.

Return the venison to the pot and cover. Bring to a boil, then drop to a low simmer and cook for 60 minutes. At this point check and adjust any seasonings or liquid as needed. Cook for 40 more minutes. You should be able to break the meat up into bite-size pieces with a wooden spoon. Then add the corn and chickpeas and cook for 10 to 20 minutes.

I like to serve this dish with grated sharp cheddar cheese, sour cream, and chopped tomatoes and radishes (both the radish root and the greens) for optional toppings.

Narrative: Brings gentleness and the desire to work toward togetherness in relationships. Promotes an understanding of the root of any difficulties being experienced, coupled with an appreciation of why it's not productive to hold on to discordant energies any longer. Ushers true warmth back into the relationship.

You might serve this dish when you've hit an emotional impasse in your relationship, and both sides (or one) has dug in their heels and emotional growth has stopped and cold distance is the norm. Or eat it if you would just like to amplify the energy of warmth and togetherness in your relationship.

CREATIVITY

🌿 Simple Purple Dead Nettle Pesto

1 cup purple dead nettles, leaves and flowering
   tops only
1 cup arugula, tightly packed
2 large bulbs garlic, cut in half
½ cup toasted almonds
½ cup extra-virgin olive oil
⅓ cup grated parmesan cheese or hemp seeds
Salt and ground black pepper to taste

Blend all the ingredients until smooth.

Narrative: This expressive pesto teaches the art of versatility, agility of mind, and the ability to mine your deepest levels of thought and express them eloquently.

You might serve this sauce when you or someone you love has a public speaking engagement or is in the process of writing—or to keep dinner party conversation lively and flowing freely!

🌿 *Jicama and Fennel Salad*

1 fennel bulb
1 medium jicama bulb, peeled and julienned
Juice of 1 lemon and 1 lime
About 2 tablespoons (more or less to your taste) of
    chopped fresh basil
1 tablespoon extra-virgin olive oil, to which you
    add a large pinch of cayenne pepper
Salt and ground black pepper to taste (start very
    lightly and taste as you go)

This salad benefits from very little seasoning due to the fresh, watery taste of jicama, which is joined with the mild licorice taste of the fennel bulb. You'll want the naturally refreshing flavors of this salad to shine through.

Adjust a mandoline to the thinnest setting. Trim the base of the fennel bulb and then halve and core it. Position one fennel half base-side down on the mandoline. Using a fluid motion, slide the fennel back and forth across the blade, allowing the shavings to fall on the cutting board. Keep going until the fennel becomes difficult to hold.

Mix all the ingredients and chill before serving.

Narrative: For those weary of life, when your creative imagination and energy are drained, this dish brings a burst of new energy, alerting you to new possibilities that are open to you now. It invites you to start afresh, make new plans, hatch new ideas, and open to the rising inspiration that is present right now.

You might serve this dish when your muse has fled the scene and you're in a creative rut or have writer's block. It's equally effective if you feel like your life has stagnated and you would like to invite fresh energy in, reengaging in life in a more exuberant manner.

🌿 Shredded Chicken Salad with Barley and Pomegranate

2 large chicken breasts
1 or 2 fresh rosemary sprigs
2 teaspoons fresh sage
4 black peppercorns
2 tablespoons Himalayan pink salt
½ teaspoon apple cider vinegar
1 cup pearled barley
2 large handfuls of arugula/rocket
½ cup pomegranate seeds
A small handful of roasted pumpkin seeds (salted or unsalted, your choice)

Dressing

¼ cup extra-virgin olive oil
¼ cup water
¼ cup white miso
1½ tablespoons rice wine vinegar
1 tablespoon brown sugar
Half a shallot, chopped

Place the chicken breasts in a pot and cover with water, then add the rosemary, sage, black peppercorns, Himalayan pink salt, and apple cider vinegar. Bring to a boil, reduce to a simmer, and cook for approximately 15 to 20 minutes. Remove, allow to cool, then shred along the grain to bite-size pieces (do not use a knife).

At the same time, cook the pearled barley according to the package directions. I suggest substituting chicken or vegetable broth for water, as it creates a richer flavor.

Set both the chicken and the cooked barley aside and allow to cool as you make the dressing, blending all the ingredients until smooth.

In a large salad bowl, combine the arugula/rocket, pomegranate seeds, pumpkin seeds, and cooled pearl barley and chicken, and toss with the dressing right before serving.

Narrative: This dish promotes discovering your unique talents and cultivates the understanding of how to share these. It brings a grounded, aware nature that allows you to synthesize your past experiences, tap into the collective unconscious, and bring this wisdom forward. This supports you to create anything and move forward with a steady, practical expression.

You might serve this dish when you lack the motivation to get started on or finish an idea or task, or if you're in a creative rut and have lost sight of who you really are and what you're capable of. It's great for polishing your unique, brilliant self to a shine and sharing these different qualities. This is also the perfect dish for a working person who splits her time between obligations and personal passions.

GOAL SETTING

✿ *Simmered Seagull Eggs with Greens*

You can substitute any type of egg in this recipe. If you can't obtain gull eggs, simply adjust the cooking time depending on the egg type and factor in the new energy signature.

> Seagull eggs
> Mayonnaise
> Chives, finely chopped
> Handful of nasturtium leaves, cut into long
>   ribbons (stack the flat leaves, roll them up tight,
>   and cut across)
> Handful of nasturtium flowers
> Handful of baby arugula/rocket
> Rice wine vinaigrette
> Celery salt

Add the eggs to a saucepan of cool water and bring to a boil. Remove from the heat, cover, and let rest for about 6 minutes, adjusting the cooking time as needed based on your altitude (see page 178). Then strain. When the eggs are cool, carefully remove their shells. Slice the rounded bottom off each egg and lightly salt; this allows you to stand them upright without them slipping.

Take a dollop of mayonnaise, add chives to taste, blend, and set aside. Add the nasturtium leaves, flowers, and arugula to a bowl, and lightly dress with the rice wine vinaigrette. On a salad plate, create a small nest of greens, using your fingers to fashion an opening in the center, where you will place one egg, topped with a small dollop of the mayonnaise and chive mixture. Finish by sprinkling with celery salt.

Narrative: Teaches the skill of turning the most unlikely things to your advantage. Stimulates ingenuity and the willingness to challenge your comfort zone, leading to endless expansion while maintaining your center and savoring life experiences.

You might serve this when you're ready to move to the next level and break your own glass ceiling, or you could serve it to someone you want to support in achieving their absolute best.

Gull's eggs are popular in England, where they've been a delicacy since the Victorian era. The gulls start building their nests at the beginning of April, and the birds lay their beautiful blue-green eggs in late April to early May. The eggs are smaller than a chicken egg, with a thinner and more delicate shell, which has a speckled pattern. The flavor of a gull's egg is much richer than a chicken egg, with a gamier taste. The rich yolks are deep orange and the whites almost creamy. Some even claim that they have a naturally mild salty taste.

Cooking Eggs at a Glance

Keep in mind that as altitude increases and atmospheric pressure decreases, the boiling point of water decreases. To compensate for the lower boiling point of water, the cooking time must be increased. Turning up the heat will not help cook food faster. No matter how high the cooking temperature, water cannot exceed its own boiling point. Depending on where you live, you may need to experiment with the following suggested cooking times.

Chicken egg (large): soft boil 3½–4 minutes; hard boil 9–10 minutes

Duck egg: soft boil 4–4½ minutes; hard boil 10–11 minutes

Emu egg: soft boil 42 minutes; hard boil 1 hour 45 minutes

Goose egg: soft boil 9–10 minutes; hard boil 13 minutes

Guinea hen egg: soft boil 4 minutes; hard boil 5–5½ minutes

Gull egg: soft boil 4½ minutes, hard boil 6 minutes

Ostrich egg: soft boil 50 minutes; hard boil 1½–2 hours

Quail egg: soft boil 30 seconds; hard boil 1 minute

Instructions for Soft- and Hard-Boiled Eggs

1. Place the egg(s) in a pot and add cold water, covering the egg(s) by 1 inch. If you are cooking multiples, make sure the eggs are in a single layer.
2. Bring to a boil over high heat.
3. As soon as the water reaches a boil, turn off the heat, cover with a snug-fitting lid, and allow to rest for the time indicated on the chart above. The exceptions are emu and ostrich eggs: keep those cooking at a low simmer until the last 20 minutes (and then remove from the heat and cover).

🌿 Niçoise Salad

Tuna steaks (1 steak per person)
Salt and ground black pepper to taste
Squeeze of lemon juice
Olive oil
Small waxy or all-purpose potatoes of choice
Green beans, ends trimmed
Eggs of choice
Lettuce of choice
Cherry tomatoes, halved
Radishes, trimmed and quartered
Black Niçoise olives
Artichoke hearts in brine

Dressing

Juice of 1 lemon
3 tablespoons white wine vinegar
1 tablespoon grainy mustard
½ cup olive oil
1 teaspoon sugar
2 tablespoons dry white wine
1 tablespoon chopped fresh thyme
Salt and fresh cracked pepper to taste

This is an incredibly fun recipe to make and there's a lot of wiggle room on the vegetables used. The key is to choose the freshest in-season ingredients that support your energetic objectives. Thinly sliced raw cucumber, fresh cooked corn, cooked asparagus, roasted mushrooms, grilled summer squash, capers, and anchovy filets can make good additions or substitutions for the ingredients listed above. Quail eggs make this a visually spectacular dish, but most often I use duck or chicken eggs.

Tuna Steaks

To cook the tuna steaks, salt and pepper both sides, squeeze a little lemon juice on top, and cook on medium-high heat in a skillet coated with a generous amount of olive oil. A typical ahi tuna steak is about 1½ inches thick. Sear on each side for about 2 minutes for medium rare (less time for rare and more time for medium). Allow to cool and then slice.

Vegetables

Scrub the potatoes and boil them in salted water with a splash of olive oil for 10 to 13 minutes, or until tender and pierced easily with a fork. Cut the potatoes into quarters or in half, depending on their size.

Cook the green beans in salted water with a splash of olive oil until tender but still very crisp, about 2 minutes. The minute you drain them, place them in an ice-water bath to stop the cooking process.

Cover the eggs with cool water and bring to a rolling boil, then turn the heat down to medium-high and cook for the appropriate amount of time depending on the egg type and desired doneness (see the chart on page 178). Cool, remove the shells, and cut in half.

Whisk together the dressing ingredients until smooth and toss the salad greens with a bit of the dressing—you don't want them saturated; the majority of the dressing should be drizzled on top after the salad is assembled so that those items are not dry. Plate the greens, arranging the vegetables, eggs, and tuna in small individual mounds on top. Drizzle dressing over each plate before serving.

Narrative: This recipe gifts the ability to move steadily along in life and uncover your secret resources, thus creating stability and financial security in your life. Doing this gives you the freedom to dream, fantasize, and be adventuresome. This kind of energy fosters creativity and the fulfillment of desires coming from your authentic self, and it teaches perseverance in the face of obstacles so you can learn your life lessons with as much ease as possible. It gifts future sight, telepathy, clairvoyance, and the ability to use these gifts for healing, often resulting in practical solutions for everyday problems. It also helps you ground yourself on the earthly plane, ultimately allowing you to thrive.

You might serve this dish anytime you (or someone else) need empowerment and support to stay on your path. It is fantastic for problem solving and encourages you to be a dreamer and to use practical, steady steps to manifest your dreams so that your deepest desires can be the bedrock of your life.

🌿 *Four Pepper Tacos*

1 red bell pepper

1 yellow bell pepper

1 Anaheim pepper

1 poblano pepper

½ teaspoon salt

¼ teaspoon ground black pepper

1½ pounds whole pork loin

3 tablespoons high-heat oil of choice

1 yellow onion

2 tablespoons dried oregano

1 tablespoon ground cumin

2 teaspoons chili powder

8 cloves garlic, smashed and cut into slivers

14.5-ounce can peeled and chopped tomatoes

1 cup chicken broth

½ cup salsa

Corn tortillas and additional toppings of choice

A Note on Cooking Oils

The Sanskrit term for oil, *sneha*, means "fat" as well as "lavish love." Oils are lubricating and fortifying; they build tissues and soothe bodily membranes. They add a rich sensuousness to our food. To discover the energetics of your chosen cooking oil—be it avocado, corn, grapeseed, peanut, sesame, or sunflower—look up the description of the plant it comes from in chapter 1.

Grill the peppers until the skin blisters, then cool, rub off the blackened skin, remove the seeds, and slice. Put aside. Salt and pepper the pork liberally and sear on both sides in the oil in a pan. Remove the pork and add the onion and spices to the pan, scraping up any brown bits. Cook until the onion softens, then add to the pan the garlic and sauté for 2 minutes. Add the peppers and tomatoes and cook for 5 minutes. Add the chicken broth and pork, cover, and cook for 30 minutes. Add the salsa and cook for another 30 minutes. Remove from the heat and let sit for 5 minutes, covered, then break up the pork with a wooden spoon. Serve on corn tortillas with additional toppings that specifically support the goals you are working on.

Narrative: This recipe gives you the ability to be a cauldron unto yourself, where you can hold and simmer everything you want to grow. This imparts inner strength, resilience, and the ability to "try, try again" until success is had, while lessening the fear of stepping into the unknown. It opens you to your wildness, to being untrammeled and not caring what others think of you. This sense of being natural allows you to grow the authentic aspects of yourself so you can follow the goals that truly nurture you. It helps you understand when you should boldly and passionately follow your dreams and when waiting in stillness for an opportunity to come to you is best.

You might serve this dish to help you understand and use the art of divine timing so you can bring your heart's desire into fruition, or to help another person in this same way. It is also dynamic for exploring your feral self, that part of you not defined by outside sources.

LETTING YOUR LIGHT SHINE

🌿 *Whole Roasted Garlic*

Garlic
Olive oil
Herbs (optional)
Sea salt (optional)

Take as many heads of garlic as you like and peel off most of the papery, outer layers, leaving the head intact with all the cloves connected. Trim about ¼ inch off the top of the head of garlic to expose the tops of the garlic cloves.

Preheat the oven to 325°F. Place the garlic in a small baking dish and drizzle the exposed tops with 1 to 2 teaspoons of olive oil. If needed, make a nest out of parchment paper to keep the cloves upright. I like to sprinkle the garlic with herbs, like rosemary or thyme, for additional depth of flavor. Cover the baking dish and bake for 35 to 40 minutes. Remove from the oven, and when the garlic is cool enough to handle, squeeze the cloves from their coverings, smash them to the desired texture, and add olive oil to taste. A pinch of sea salt is optional.

Narrative: Amplifies the divine light that dwells in your core, bringing warmth and receptivity and fostering the energy of inclusiveness and true caring. Supports respecting the freedom of those you love, teaching by example, and holding space for others to find their way without pushing them along before they're ready.

You might serve this dish to hold space for someone when they're in an emotional or spiritual growth spurt to help them anchor their newly acquired understandings, allowing them to feel completely adored and nourished while in the process.

🌿 Rustic Pearl Barley and Roasted Vegetable Salad

½ cup pearl barley
1½ cups water or vegetable broth
Avocado oil
Salt
1 large jewel yam
2 large parsnips
2 large carrots
½ white onion
Ground black pepper
Garlic powder, to taste
4 stalks fresh thyme
Honey, to taste
2 teaspoons white miso
3 tablespoons chopped scallions
2 cloves garlic, smashed
¼ cup full-fat plain yogurt
Mixed fresh herbs, roasted pumpkin seeds, and/or
    pomegranate seeds, for garnish (optional)

Barley

Combine the barley with the water or broth, 1 teaspoon avocado oil, and 1 teaspoon salt in a medium pot. Bring to a boil, reduce the heat, cover, and cook for 45 to 60 minutes. Taste after 45 minutes—you want a semifirm texture for the barley.

Vegetables

Peel the vegetables and cut into bite-size pieces. Line a baking sheet with parchment paper or spread a very thin layer of oil on the sheet for easier cleanup. Spread the vegetables out evenly and drizzle with avocado oil. Sprinkle with salt, pepper, garlic powder to taste, and thyme (removed from the stalks), drizzle with honey, then stir to coat the vegetables. Place in an oven that's been preheated to 375°F. Cook for 30 minutes, then stir and cook for another 15 to 30 minutes, depending on how caramelized you like your vegetables.

Dressing

Combine in a blender the white miso, chopped scallions (white and green parts), garlic cloves, 4 to 6 tablespoons avocado oil, yogurt, and water as needed. Blend until smooth and rich.

Place the cooked barley in a large mixing bowl and toss with half of the dressing. Add the roasted vegetables and the remainder of the dressing and gently fold in. You may want to garnish with mixed fresh herbs, roasted pumpkin seeds, and/or pomegranate seeds.

Narrative: Helpful for exploring the bright, luminous gifts that are unique to each person, and bringing them to the surface to be explored and cultivated. Wonderful for self-expression and for learning that each person's gift set is unique and valuable. Supports not judging your self-worth based on comparing yourself to others, but to celebrate your authenticity and how you incarnated.

You might serve this dish if you or someone else is ready to explore a deeper layer of the self and what you have to offer this world, having it be an open-ended question that you have not pre-answered. It can be beneficial if you are stuck in a pattern of defining your self-worth based on comparing yourself to others' accomplishments or patterning yourself after another person at the expense of being your authentic self.

DECISION-MAKING

🌿 Roasted Carrots with Carrot Greens Chimichurri

1 bunch carrots with greens intact
2 cloves garlic, chopped
3 green onions, white and green parts, chopped
Good-quality extra-virgin olive oil
¼ cup white vinegar
Salt and freshly ground black pepper
3 teaspoons bruised dried oregano
2 pinches crushed red pepper flakes

Prepare the chimichurri sauce first, allowing the flavors to meld as the carrots roast.

Chimichurri Sauce

Remove any fibrous bits from the carrot greens; wash and squeeze out the excess moisture. Roughly chop the greens, combine them in a food processor with the garlic and green onions, and process until very fine. Place carrot greens mixture in a bowl; add ½ cup olive oil, white vinegar, 1 to 2 teaspoons salt (to taste), ½ teaspoon pepper, oregano, and red pepper flakes. Allow to sit for at least 30 minutes.

Basic Roasted Carrots

Leave the peel on the carrots and give them a sound scrubbing. I like to leave the slender filament on the tip, as it crisps up wonderfully. Have a glass roasting pan at the ready. Using your hands, thoroughly rub olive oil all over the carrots, place in the pan, and sprinkle with salt and pepper. Roast uncovered for 20 to 30 minutes at 425°F or until tender.

To serve, drizzle chimichurri sauce on top of the carrots, with a small dish of the sauce on the side.

Narrative: Offers support if you tend to overanalyze, overworry, and get caught up in "what ifs" to the point of personal detriment. Helps you be in the here and now and feel safe while doing so. Assists you in finding your center, standing firm, and acting from a place of strength.

You might serve this dish when you feel paralyzed and can't make a decision. This energy allows you to feel into your options, take a deep breath, and make choices based on what's truly best for you, without fear.

🌿 Garlic-Scented Hedgehog Mushroom and Asparagus Sauté

About 1 pound hedgehog mushrooms
About ½ pound chanterelle mushrooms
Olive oil as needed
Butter as needed
½ pound asparagus, cut into small pieces
3 Roma tomatoes, chopped, seeds removed
2 sprigs fresh thyme
3 cloves garlic, minced
2 tablespoons or so dry white wine
Fleur de sel finishing salt
Freshly ground black pepper

Clean the mushrooms with a mushroom brush or a damp paper towel (avoid rinsing mushrooms in water if at all possible) and trim the ends. Heat the butter and oil in a large sauté pan over medium-high heat, add the mushrooms, and sauté, stirring occasionally, until the mushrooms release their liquid. As they start to brown, add the asparagus, tomatoes, and thyme, and cook for about 5 minutes. Then add the garlic and wine, and continue to cook, scraping up any brown bits, until the liquid has evaporated. Remove from the heat and season with salt and pepper to taste. If you kept the thyme on its stalk, remove it now.

Narrative: Helps you to not act in haste, providing you with the patience to penetrate deeply into the heart of the matter, expanding your subtle perception so you can more clearly see energetic information from other people. This allows you to carefully consider motives and circumstances (yours and theirs) before taking action.

Although there is no circumstance in which this dish is not helpful, you might serve it whenever you're trying to navigate another person you're puzzled by, especially when you're making decisions that will affect not only you but the other person. It supports you in trying to understand where someone is coming from so you don't react in a judgmental way and can thereby apply empathy to the situation. In short, this dish can help you understand your environment in a clear manner and see other people's motivations and the best way to respond.

Often most of us have no idea why we behave the way we do. When you don't understand your own or someone else's behavior and why you or they are triggered, this dish can help you see things more clearly, with greater insight, so you can then apply compassion to the situation and formulate the best response.

🌿 *Pork Spare Ribs with Blackberry Barbecue Sauce*

Barbecue Sauce

> 3 cups fresh blackberries
> ¼ cup brown sugar
> ½ cup ketchup
> ½ teaspoon onion powder
> ½ teaspoon garlic powder
> ½ teaspoon paprika (California sweet)
> ½ teaspoon chili powder
> 1 tablespoon ginger powder
> 2 tablespoons apple cider vinegar
> ⅓ cup Trappey's Spicy Hot Cayenne Pepper Sauce
> (or Tabasco or your personal favorite cayenne
> pepper sauce)
> 2 tablespoons Worcestershire sauce
> 4 tablespoons salted butter, cubed
> 1 tablespoon ground black pepper

Pork Spare Ribs
Pork ribs
Salt and freshly ground black pepper

Sauce Preparation

Blend the blackberries in a food processor until smooth, then strain through a fine-mesh strainer. Return the berries to the food processor with all the other ingredients and pulse until blended. Add to a medium saucepan and cook for about 5 minutes over medium heat, stirring often, until thickened. Set aside and allow the flavors to mellow.

Pork Rib Preparation

Most store-bought ribs have what's known as "silverskin," a thin membrane over the underside of the ribs. Unless you just love wielding a knife, ask your butcher to remove it for you. Next, boil the pork until the ribs are slightly soft but not falling apart, about 25 minutes, or cook them in a pressure cooker for about 8 minutes. Remove the ribs and season liberally with salt and pepper or a dry rub of your choice. At this stage the ribs are semicooked, so you'll want to finish them off on an oiled grill. My preferred way to grill ribs is with a rib rack. Brush the barbecue sauce on both sides of the ribs, place on the rack, and grill over medium heat for 10 to 15 minutes on each side, applying barbecue sauce as needed to keep the ribs moist and juicy, and checking for doneness as you go. When the meat begins to pull away from the ends of the bones, pierce it with a fork, and if the tines slip easily through the ribs, you're ready to serve. Have extra barbecue sauce on the side.

Narrative: Helps strengthens the ability to act decisively from a clear sense of what you want and who you are, without sacrificing any aspects you deem important, as you move forward toward your goals. Also offers the perspective of a wide overview.

You might serve this dish when you feel boxed in and stymied when working toward a goal. When you know where you want to end up but are not sure how to get there, this vibration will help clarify your direction and help you create a plan of action.

EMOTIONAL SUPPORT

🌿 *Chilled Cucumber and Avocado Soup*

1 English cucumber
1 large ripe avocado
2 green onions
½ cup full-fat plain yogurt
½ cup buttermilk
1 teaspoon salt
½ teaspoon ground black pepper
A dash or two of ground cayenne pepper
Sliced radishes, chopped herbs, and feta cheese, for garnish

Dice the cucumber and avocado and slice the green onions. Reserve half of the sliced green parts of the green onions for a garnish. Combine the rest of the green onions, cucumber, and avocado in a blender. Add the yogurt, buttermilk, and spices to the blender and blend until smooth. Adjust the seasoning to taste.

Offer thinly sliced radishes, the reserved green onion leaves mixed with chopped herbs of choice, and feta cheese to sprinkle on top of this cold soup. I like to provide Kilauea Onyx black sea salt and Molokai red sea salt at the table.

Narrative: Eases difficult emotional states, harmonizes the body and mind by dissolving tension, and offers shelter when you're feeling overwhelmed with emotion or by life events.

You might serve this dish when you or someone else received some unsettling news or experienced a shocking personal event, or you're just tired and worn down by life and in need of a reboot.

🌱 Radish Leaf Salad Dressing

Leafy tops from 1 bunch radishes, trimmed and
    washed
⅓ bunch of parsley, trimmed and washed
3 tablespoons white vinegar
½ cup toasted shelled pumpkin seeds
1 or 2 lemons, juiced
2 pinches red pepper flakes
⅓ cup extra-virgin olive oil
1 or 2 cloves garlic, crushed

Add all the ingredients to your blender and blend until smooth. Add water until you achieve your desired consistency. Taste and adjust the seasonings.

Narrative: Promotes a strong sense of individuality and celebrating what makes you unique rather than feeling isolated by it.

You might serve this dressing when you or someone you care for is feeling awkward or misunderstood in personal expression. It will help you bathe in the light of *you* and foster deep self-appreciation.

🌿 Avocado and Lime Shrimp Salad

¼ cup chopped red onion
3 limes, juiced
1 teaspoon extra-virgin olive oil
Salt and freshly ground black pepper to taste
1 pound cooked shrimp, peeled, deveined, and
    chopped
1 medium tomato, diced, seeds removed
1 jalapeño pepper, seeds removed, finely diced
1 tablespoon chopped cilantro
Ripe avocado(s)

Combine the red onion, two-thirds of the lime juice, olive oil, salt, and pepper; let rest for at least 5 minutes, allowing the flavors to blend.

In another bowl, combine the chopped shrimp, tomato, jalapeño, cilantro, and salt and pepper to taste, and gently toss before mixing in the marinated red onions.

Cut the avocado(s) in half and remove the pit to make a "bowl" in the center. Squeeze a little lime juice on each side and sprinkle with salt. Spoon the shrimp mixture into the avocado bowls and serve.

Narrative: Allows you to maintain your inherent innocence and sweetness and not be jaded when being jostled around in this complicated world.

You might try serving this dish if you feel like you're bogged down by the weight of the world and find you have a short fuse due to emotional fatigue.

❦ Watercress with Warm Wild Mushrooms

3 to 4 tablespoons extra-virgin olive oil
½ pound chanterelle mushrooms, whole
½ pound hedgehog mushrooms, whole
½ pound lobster mushrooms, if very large cut to
*   match other mushrooms' size*
Coarse salt and freshly ground black pepper
4 cloves garlic, chopped
2 teaspoons minced fresh thyme
3 cups fresh watercress, tough stems removed
4 tablespoons vinaigrette of choice (I like balsamic)

Heat the olive oil in a large pan over medium heat. Working in batches, add the mushrooms, season with salt and pepper to taste, and sauté for about 5 minutes or until the mushrooms have softened and exuded their liquid and the pan is almost dry. Remove from the heat and stir in the garlic and thyme. Taste, and if necessary, season with additional salt and pepper. Using a slotted spoon, transfer the mushrooms to a colander placed in a mixing bowl and drain. There should be no juices left if cooked correctly.

Place the clean, trimmed watercress in a large mixing bowl. Add the warm mushrooms and drizzle with just enough vinaigrette to season lightly. Apply salt and pepper to taste and toss to blend. Serve immediately.

Narrative: When you're feeling overstimulated by ordinary daily events, this recipe facilitates the ability to partake in life without being swept away by the multitude of dizzying aspects that flow through your day. It allows you to firmly ground yourself, take a breath, feel solid in yourself, and condense the information all around you into usable, manageable bits.

You might serve this dish when your life is so harried you don't know which end is up, and you see no end in sight. This recipe will create an island of repose where you can catch your breath and filter what is required of you in order of importance, allowing you to know what to move on and what to put on the back burner, creating a more manageable day. This dish tonifies the energetic body and offsets fatigue that sleep alone cannot quench.

🌿 Avocado Toast with Radish Leaf Vinaigrette and Microgreens

1 bunch radishes with fresh, vibrant leaves
4 tablespoons avocado oil, plus more for drizzling
    on the avocado and brushing on the toast
2 tablespoons champagne vinegar
1½ teaspoons smooth Dijon mustard
2 tablespoons water
1 clove garlic
Salt and freshly ground black pepper to taste
1 ripe avocado
1 or 2 lemon wedges
¼ teaspoon garlic powder
Pinch of thyme
Dash of cayenne pepper
1 slice thick rustic bread
Radish microgreens or sprouts

Vinaigrette

Wash the radishes and break off the leaves. Rip those leaves into rough pieces and put them in a food processer, to which you add the avocado oil, vinegar, mustard, water, garlic clove, salt, and pepper. Blend until smooth. Season to your delight.

Avocado

Split the avocado, remove the pit with a spoon, and scoop the flesh into a bowl. Add a drizzle of avocado oil, a squeeze of one or two lemon wedges, the garlic powder, a large pinch of thyme, and a dash of cayenne pepper. Mash coarsely, and season with salt and pepper to taste.

Microgreen Topping

Slice the radishes paper-thin. Take a handful of the washed radish microgreens or sprouts—enough to fit nicely in the center of the bread—place them in a bowl with 5 to 10 pieces of radish. Toss with a small amount of vinaigrette.

Toast

I highly recommend thick-sliced rustic bread with a good bite. Brush the slices lightly with avocado oil and place on the open rack of your oven on broil. Keep an eye out, and once the bread slices have browned nicely, remove them. Spread the avocado evenly over the toast and drizzle with the vinaigrette, making a beautiful nest with the microgreens on top.

Narrative: This dish is a powerful vibration when working with addiction, be it to a substance, sex, anger, or any other kind of behavior. It clears the underlying causes that started the cycle and brings powerful healing energy into your cellular memory and calcified energy tracts that engage the craving for the substance or behavior that's causing you harm.

You might serve this dish (with a big helping of compassion) to yourself or anyone in need of support and love.

🌿 Ricotta-Stuffed Squash Blossoms

1 cup whole-milk ricotta cheese
1 teaspoon finely chopped fresh thyme
Zest of 1 lemon
½ teaspoon lemon juice
½ teaspoon ground mace
2 pinches ground cayenne pepper
1 teaspoon sea salt
½ teaspoon ground white pepper
2 eggs
Squash blossoms (approx. 3 per person for an appetizer)
1 cup flour
Grapeseed oil
Finishing salt

Using a wooden spoon, mix the ricotta with the thyme, lemon zest and juice, mace, cayenne, salt, and pepper until smooth. Add to a pastry (piping) bag fitted with a large plain tip. In another bowl, beat 2 eggs.

Remove the stamens from the blossoms. Pipe about 1 tablespoon of the cheese mixture into each blossom, then roll the filled blossom in all-purpose flour, dip in the egg mixture, and roll in the flour again, shaking off any excess.

Add a heavy layer of oil to a deep-sided frying pan and heat until it reaches 375°F. Fry a few blossoms at a time (take care not to overcrowd them), turning once, until golden brown, about 3 to 4 minutes.

Transfer to a paper towel–lined plate and sprinkle with fleur de sel finishing salt (or something similar). Keep the blossoms in a warm oven at 200°F until ready to serve.

Narrative: For prickly people who are always annoyed by something, this dish will help soothe how you perceive the world and will aid you in not finding other people and circumstances so irritating. On the other hand, if you are in a situation where you have to communicate with a prickly person, squash blossoms will take the edge off during this exchange, allowing you to stay calm and centered, without personal defenses going up.

You might serve this dish before heading into a tough situation, knowing the other party is difficult and may act in an irrational manner that you cannot anticipate. If you yourself are the prickly one, this recipe will help you smooth your quills, allowing you to interact with others in a more peaceable manner.

🌿 Fragrant Chicken Thighs with Green Chickpeas, Carrots, and Zucchini

2 chicken thighs, skin and fat removed
¼ cup sea salt
High-heat oil of choice
1 teaspoon finely minced fresh ginger
1 teaspoon ground turmeric
1 teaspoon curry powder
1 teaspoon ground coriander
½ teaspoon ground cumin
¼ teaspoon ground cardamom
¼ teaspoon ground mustard seed
¼ teaspoon ground cayenne pepper
3 bay leaves
¼ teaspoon ground black pepper
1 teaspoon brown sugar
4 tablespoons ghee, plus more as needed
1 medium yellow onion, coarsely chopped
6 cloves garlic, smashed and sliced
8 ounces tomato sauce
2 tablespoons flour
1½ cups chicken broth
½ cup milk or coconut milk
3 large carrots, peeled and cut into large chunks
1¼ cups green chickpeas,* defrosted if frozen
1 large zucchini, scrubbed and cut into large chunks

*A green chickpea is simply a normal garbanzo bean that's been harvested while immature and still in its green state, full of moisture and color. Green chickpeas don't need to be reconstituted with water, and they usually come frozen or fresh in the shell.

Chicken Preparation

Cover the chicken thighs with cold water, add ¼ cup sea salt, and stir to dissolve the salt. Let soak for 30 minutes. Then remove the thighs from the bath, pat dry with paper towels, rub with oil on both sides, and sprinkle liberally with pepper. Grill for 5 minutes on each side (if you don't have a grill available, sear the thighs in a pan on each side for 5 minutes) and then set aside.

Spice Bath and Other Bits

Add the spices and sugar to a deep-sided pan and warm for 2 minutes, then add the ghee and heat for 1 minute, stirring constantly. Add the onion and sauté until it starts to soften, then add the garlic and cook, stirring constantly, for 2 minutes. Add the tomato sauce. Cook for 3 minutes, then add the flour and additional ghee, if needed, stirring for about 3 minutes. Slowly stir in the chicken broth and cook for 3 minutes, then add the milk and cook for 1 minute. Add the chicken thighs and carrot chunks and cook for 30 minutes with the lid on. Flip the chicken thighs and cook for another 15 minutes, then add the green chickpeas and cook for 15 more minutes, lid on. Remove from the heat, remove the bay leaves, add the zucchini, stir gently, and allow to sit for 10 minutes before serving. I suggest serving on rice.

For a vegetarian alternative to this dish, switch out the protein. Instead of using chicken, you might try pressed tofu; see below.

Variation: Pressed Tofu

To press tofu, sandwich your whole extra-firm tofu block between dish towels (waffle-weave towels work best) or paper towels. Place a flat surface on the top and bottom, such as a cutting board or baking sheet, and weigh it down with heavy item(s), such as canned goods or cookbooks. Let the tofu sit for at least 30 minutes. Change the towels if they become too moist. Cut the tofu into cubes after the pressing process is complete.

Narrative: Difficulties do not just vanish because we will them to. Ultimately we all have to face whatever daunting energy is holding us back and address it directly, no matter how frightening it is, finding the strength to move forward. Only then can we allow new outcomes into life. This recipe will fortify you and give you the strength to face challenges head-on, with a clear mind and open eyes, ultimately allowing you to resolve the situation at hand.

You might serve this dish when you reach a cusp and are afraid to push forward into uncharted territory, be it work, spirituality, relationship, and so forth. It's also helpful when you're mired and know you need a change of perspective, or for working with longstanding aggregates that are deeply ingrained in your energetic body that create behaviors and/or situations that have ensnared you.

CELEBRATION OF LIFE, FAMILY, AND COMMUNITY

🌿 Cumin-Scented Grilled Corn on the Cob

Desired number of ears of corn, husks still on
4 tablespoons salted butter
½ teaspoon ground cumin
¼ teaspoon chili powder
1 lime, juiced
Pinch of sugar
Salt and ground black pepper to taste

Leaving the husks attached, remove the silk and rinse the corn. Gently put the husks back in place, then soak the corn cobs in water for at least 30 minutes (the corn needs to be completely covered in water). Bring the butter to room temperature and whip in the cumin, chili powder, lime juice, sugar, salt, and black pepper. Remove the corn from the water and carefully peel down the husks, making sure you keep them intact, and spread the butter evenly on the corn. Put the husks back in place (they might be a little loose, but that is okay) and grill the corn, turning frequently, until the husks are charred and beginning to shrivel and the corn is tender, about 10 minutes.

This is such a forgiving recipe and not persnickety at all! Whatever temperature you're already grilling at will work. This next part is completely optional, but my favorite way to finish off this style of corn is to very carefully (so you don't burn *your fingers) peel back the husk, place the ears directly on the grill, and, depending on how hot your grill is, grill for 1 to 3 minutes, turning the corn halfway through the grilling. Basically you're looking for a nice char.*

Narrative: Helps you open to enjoying the sensual pleasures of being on this Earth. Gently opens you up to appreciate all the wonders life has to offer so you can create your own paradise in the here and now.

You might serve this dish when you want to amplify the pleasures of being alive, allowing you to take life in deeply and savor your experiences.

❦ Duck Dippy Eggs with Asparagus Soldiers

> 1 bunch asparagus
> Salt and freshly ground black pepper
> Extra-virgin olive oil
> Butter (optional)
> Garlic powder
> 2 duck eggs
> White vinegar
> Johnny-jump-up petals
> Chives
> Buttered toast points

Wash and break off the tough ends of the asparagus. Bring enough water to a boil in a large pan to cover the asparagus completely. Add 1 tablespoon of salt and a dash of olive oil, and cook the asparagus for 3 to 6 minutes, with the lid on, to the tenderness you desire. Drain, then immediately put the asparagus back in the pan and stir in a small amount of butter or olive oil. Lightly season with salt, pepper, and about ¼ teaspoon garlic powder and toss to mix. Put the lid back on to keep the asparagus warm.

Crack the eggs into 2 separate teacups and bring to room temperature. In a large pot, bring water to a boil, add 1 tablespoon white vinegar, and turn down to a simmer. Use a whisk to create a vortex as you slip one egg (you can cook only one at a time) gently into the center. Cook for 4 to 5 minutes (adjusting as needed for altitude) and remove with a slotted spoon and drain before you plate. Repeat to cook the second egg.

Finish the poached duck eggs with a sprinkling of finishing salt and a good grinding of fresh black pepper. Garnish with fresh Johnny-jump-ups and chives. Serve with the asparagus and buttery toast points for dipping in the poached egg yolk.

Narrative: Since duck eggs are about navigating your emotions, you can use this dish to access either the bright or heavy side of those. Asparagus allows you to address heavy emotions such as depression, feelings of abandonment, recovering from abuse, and fear. Or you can celebrate due to the Johnny-jump-ups, as they bring the bright, exciting, light, celebratory aspects of being alive. Eggs also hold the energy of new beginnings and endings of old cycles that don't feel good, so you can birth something new and wonderful.

You might serve this dish to celebrate the birth of a child, an idea, or an event when you want to revel in the wonderment of something truly new. Or you could serve this in support of ending a cycle of heaviness, either your own or someone else's, to release dense energies that hamper joy and growth. This dish is also powerful for stopping recurring thoughts that you can't simply will away.

❧ Succotash

1 cup olive oil

3 teaspoons butter

4 cloves garlic, finely chopped

1 medium white onion, chopped

2 bell peppers of your choice, seeded, deveined, and
diced

2 10-ounce packages frozen lima beans, rinsed
under warm running water and drained (or
about 2½ cups if fresh)

3 cups fresh or frozen corn kernels (approximately
4 ears)

Coarse salt and freshly ground pepper

2 medium zucchini, seeded and diced

2 tablespoons chopped fresh sage

2 tablespoons chopped fresh thyme leaves

In a large skillet, heat the oil and butter over medium-high heat, then add the garlic and onion and cook for about 4 minutes. Add the bell peppers, lima beans, and corn, season with salt and pepper, and cook, stirring occasionally, until the vegetables are semi-tender, about 5 minutes. Add the zucchini and herbs and cook for about 5 more minutes.

Narrative: This dish promotes living in a state of wonder, curiosity, and flow, taking in all the sweetness that life has to offer, allowing passion, enthusiasm, and warmth to be your driving force.

You might serve this dish anytime you need to reconnect with the succor of life and rediscover wonderment, or serve it at any festive occasion when you want to amplify the joyous feelings.

🌿 Creamy Tomato Pasta Sauce with Meat and Herbs

For my entire life, my grandmother and mother served a variation of this dish at large family dinners. This is my own interpretation, which pays homage to them both. The maple bacon is a nod to my mother, who always admonished me to add a little sugar to my sauce. She claimed it would "bring sweetness to those at the table." I love the way the subtle smoky-sweet of the bacon adds to this dish. My grandmother would have used pancetta.

2 celery stalks (tops intact if possible)
2 large carrots
1 medium white onion
3 bay leaves
6 basil leaves, chopped
2 tablespoons chopped fresh oregano
1 teaspoon salt
½ teaspoon ground black pepper
2 tablespoons olive oil
2 tablespoons butter
2 pieces thick maple bacon, cut coarsely, OR ¼ cup
    cubed pancetta
1½ pounds lean ground beef
6 cloves garlic, sliced thinly
2½ cups chopped plum tomatoes
1 cup rich beef stock
1 cup red wine
3 cups tomato sauce
2 cups whole milk
Rigatoni, pappardelle, or tagliatelle pasta
Parmesan and additional chopped fresh herbs to garnish

Chop the celery, carrots, and onion finely, about the same size. Add the herbs and chopped vegetables to a large sauté pan with deep sides and a lid. Add the salt, pepper, olive oil, and butter, and cook over medium-high heat for about 5 minutes. Cook the bacon in a separate pan until it crisps, then add it to the vegetable mix. Add the ground beef to the pan the bacon cooked in and sauté until browned—you want the meat to stick a bit to the pan. Drain the excess oil out of the pan. Add the garlic, cook for 2 minutes, then add the bacon and vegetable mixture and the chopped tomatoes, scraping the bottom of the pan. Simmer for 5 minutes. Add the beef broth and red wine. Simmer for about 10 minutes, stirring frequently. Add the tomato sauce, cover, and cook for 60 minutes. Add the milk, cover, and cook for another 45 minutes, stirring occasionally. Remove the lid and cook until the sauce has reached a rich, thick consistency.

Prepare the pasta according to the package directions. Top with pasta sauce, parmesan cheese, and additional chopped fresh herbs.

Narrative: This dish brings the energy of celebrating the family unit and strengthening family ties, coupled with the desire to understand why traditions are important to learn and pass along. It also stimulates the desire to create new traditions to be shared with generations to come.

You might serve this dish to usher in nostalgia and encourage storytelling, especially among the older generation. If you're drawn to being the recordkeeper in your family, this vibration is helpful for exploring family genealogy. It can help the new generations navigate the family lines—not only to celebrate the family's past, but also to build on that and create new traditions to be cherished and passed down.

SENSUAL PLEASURES

🌿 Blistered Padrón Peppers

> 1 pound padrón peppers
> Olive oil
> Flaky sea salt

Wash the peppers and pat them dry. Heat the olive oil in a large skillet over high heat until just smoking. Add half of the peppers; cook, tossing occasionally, until the skins are blistered and the flesh is softened, about 4 minutes. Transfer to a bowl, sprinkle liberally with salt, and toss to coat. Repeat this process with the remaining peppers. Best eaten hot.

Narrative: This recipe brings a full-blooded suggestiveness that encourages you to be physically passionate, expressive, and uninhibited.

You might want to serve this dish before going dancing, to a party, or on date night.

🌿 Roasted Cornish Game Hens with Elephant Garlic

> 2 Cornish game hens, skin removed
> Salt and lemon pepper to taste
> ¼ cup olive oil
> 8 tablespoons salted butter
> 3 tablespoons lemon juice
> 2 sprigs fresh rosemary
> 1 head elephant garlic (remove the papery outer
>   skin but leave the layer closest to the bulb intact
>   and separate each clove)
> 1 cinnamon stick
> 2 whole cardamom pods
> Zest of 1 orange
> 1 tablespoon orange juice
> 2½ cups whole milk
> 2 tablespoons cornstarch

Liberally salt and lemon-pepper the game hens, inside and out. Heat the olive oil and 4 tablespoons of the butter in a large pan over medium-high heat. Add the game hens and brown for about 3 minutes on each side. Remove the game hens, sprinkle lemon juice inside the cavities, and place 1 rosemary sprig in each, then truss the legs with kitchen twine. Using the leftover oil and butter mixture, briefly cook the garlic, cinnamon, and cardamom pods over medium-high heat for about 2 minutes.

Place the game hens in a roasting pan, breast side up. Add the orange zest and juice and the garlic, cinnamon, and cardamom pods, placing the garlic on the side so it will be submerged in the cooking liquid. Then add the milk (do not pour directly on the hens). Finish by cutting the remaining 4 tablespoons butter into small pieces and placing them directly on the breasts. Bake at 375°F for 90 minutes.

Once the birds are finished, allow the garlic to cool and then squeeze the cloves from their skins and mash them together. This makes a beautiful roasted garlic paste. The cooking liquid will have curdled due to the citrus and milk, so, using a slotted spoon, remove the soft curdles of milk and set them aside. Fish out the whole herbs and spices, and bring the rest of the cooking liquid back to simmer.

Mix the cornstarch with a little cold water in a liquid measuring cup and stir until very smooth to make a slurry. Slowly add 1 cup of the hot liquid from the roasting pan to the slurry, stirring the entire time. Once it is thoroughly blended, add the slurry to the simmering liquid and stir for about 1 minute, until thickened.

To serve: Plate your game hen, drizzle with gravy (do not smother), and top with the curdled milk, offering the roasted garlic on the side. Pass the additional gravy around the table.

Narrative: Brings out your hidden desires, dissolves frustrations, fosters feelings of contentment, brings the energy of bliss and growth, and amplifies lovemaking and teaches how to use this sacred energy to invoke fertility and abundance (in any form required). Ultimately allows you to bask in a warm glow of happiness.

You might serve this dish to your beloved to celebrate your love for him/her/them and enhance the loving feelings that already exist. Or you could serve it at a start of a new relationship to help foster its growth into something strong and beautiful. It is also very powerful to mindfully eat as a couple when you're starting a new project or venture together and want to bless it. Of course, you can just tap into the energy of being contented, bliss-filled, and creative, without the sexual element, if that's more appropriate for the occasion.

🌱 Rabbit Ragu with Dried Mushrooms and Pappardelle

I grew up eating rabbit due to my father raising them, and my mother being the resourceful soul she is, I have eaten rabbit many different ways. One of my favorites is the following ragu.* The earthiness of the mushrooms paired with the strong presence of herbs gives this dish a nice "forest floor" taste that pairs easily with rabbit.

¼ cup dried porcini mushrooms
1 large whole rabbit, cut into pieces (ask your
    butcher to do it if you don't know how)
Salt and ground pepper to taste
All-purpose flour
Olive oil
2 cups finely chopped red onion
½ pound cremini mushrooms, chopped
1 cup minced carrot
1 cup minced celery
4 tablespoons minced garlic
3 cups grassy sauvignon blanc
1 cup chopped and peeled canned tomatoes with juice
2 bay leaves
3 sprigs fresh thyme
1 sprig fresh rosemary
1 teaspoon crushed red pepper flakes

*Ragu is a class of Italian pasta sauces made with ground, minced, or shredded meat, vegetables, and occasionally tomatoes.

1 teaspoon dried oregano
1 cup chicken broth
Pappardelle pasta
Butter
Parmesan cheese, finely grated
Fresh flat-leaf parsley, chopped
Crushed red pepper flakes, to taste

Soak the porcini mushrooms in hot water for 20 minutes, reserving the liquid. Slice into ribbons or keep whole, depending on your personal preference.

Season the rabbit pieces with salt and pepper and dredge them in flour, then brown in small batches in medium-hot olive oil in a large Dutch oven for about 3 minutes per side. Remove and place on a paper towel–lined plate.

Using the same oil (you many need to add more), turn the heat down to medium-low; pay attention and set the heat even lower if needed, as this needs to be a slow cook to caramelize properly. Add the onion, mushrooms (both types), carrot, and celery to the pot and cook for about 20 minutes, until the vegetables are caramelized. Next add the garlic, wine, 3 tablespoons of the reserved mushroom liquid, tomatoes, and all the herbs and spices, and simmer for about 15 minutes. Return the rabbit to the pot, add the chicken broth, and bring to a boil. Immediately reduce the heat to a simmer, cover, and cook for about 1½ hours. Your goal is fall-off-the-bone tenderness. Remove the rabbit from the sauce and let cool, and then remove the meat from the bones and shred with your fingers into bite-size pieces. Return only the meat to the sauce. Fish out the bay leaves and thyme and rosemary stalks and add salt and pepper to taste.

Bring a large pot of salted water to a boil, add the pappardelle, and cook according to the package directions until al dente. Drain the pasta and toss in some butter, just enough to coat.

Serve the ragu over the hot cooked pasta, garnished with grated parmesan cheese, fresh flat-leaf parsley, and red pepper flakes.

Narrative: Helps you explore the essence of love that grows out of being in union with a beloved. Encourages whispering sweet nothings and words of kindness, and expressing your affection through touch and softness of action. If either party is timid or hesitant, this dish will allow them to radiate out all they are in their completeness, as they feel safe to do so in the presence of the other. This facilitates each person sharing themself to the fullest.

You might want to serve this dish if the object of your affection has come from a previously difficult relationship and is gun-shy and needs additional support to feel safe so they can be fully present in a relationship. It's a dynamic dish to serve to someone you care for if you feel it would benefit them and enhance their life to learn the language of love. If you yourself have a complicated romantic history, eating this dish will help you open up for a new relationship, so you don't carry old baggage into it.

ENHANCING YOUR SPIRITUAL WORK

❧ *Marbled Goose Tea Eggs*

Rich and creamy goose eggs are roughly the equivalent of two hen's eggs. One per person as a tea snack or appetizer is generally enough.

> Goose eggs
> 8 black tea bags
> 2 tablespoons black peppercorns
> 2 star anise pods
> 8 whole cloves
> Zest and juice of 1 orange
> 1 teaspoon kosher salt
> Greens of choice
> 3 tablespoons goji berries, softened in tea for about
>   5 minutes, until plump and juicy
> Soy sauce or salt for dipping

In a large saucepan, cover the eggs with 2 inches of water and bring to a boil. Remove the pan from the heat, cover, and let stand for about 13 minutes for a hard-boiled egg. Using a slotted spoon, transfer the eggs to a work surface. Tap the eggs all over with the back of a spoon to crack the shells. To the saucepan in which you cooked the eggs, immediately add the tea bags, peppercorns, anise pods, cloves, orange zest and juice, and salt, stirring to dissolve the salt. Then add the eggs, cover, and refrigerate overnight.

Drain and peel the eggs and nest them on a bed of greens (mizuna greens are a nice choice, either cold or prepared in a simple sauté) and sprinkle with goji berries softened in tea. Serve with a side of soy sauce or salt for dipping.

Narrative: This recipe is pure creativity, the knowing that springs from the luminous mind, which helps you make discoveries that lie dormant deep within. It provides a gateway to your own akashic records for self-instruction.

You might serve this when you need to stimulate your intuitive body or when you seek access to the akashic records, are trying to puzzle something out, or are studying in earnest and need help assimilating the information.

❧ *Puree of Pumpkin Soup in Sugar Pumpkin Tureens*

2 cups pumpkin puree
3 quarts vegetable stock
1½ cups half-and-half
1½ cups whole milk
4 cloves garlic, minced
⅓ cup maple syrup
1½ teaspoons Chinese five-spice powder
3 tablespoons butter
Salt and pepper to taste
Pumpkin seed oil to taste
Chevre/goat cheese
Molokai red sea salt
Marigold petals
Fresh chives, chopped

The Soup

Mix the first four ingredients in a pot and bring to a boil, stirring often. Then add the garlic, maple syrup, Chinese five-spice powder, butter, salt, and pepper, give a good stir, and simmer until the flavors meld, about 15 to 20 minutes, stirring often. Adjust the seasonings to your liking.

Sugar Pumpkin Tureen

1 sugar pumpkin per person (each pumpkin will serve as a bowl; choose your preferred size accordingly)

Rinse the pumpkins, then take a paring knife and cut out a hole in the top to make the right size for eating soup. Completely remove all the seeds and as much of the stringy pulp as possible, then lightly rub the interior of the pumpkins with olive oil and sprinkle with sea salt. Bake at 350°F until the pumpkins are softened and warmed, but not mushy, about 10 to 15 minutes.

Finishing Touch

Ladle the soup into the tureens and drizzle the pumpkin seed oil in a pleasing design on top. Add the chevre and finish with cracked fresh black pepper, a sprinkling of Molokai red sea salt (this premium salt is not for cooking, just for sprinkling on top after the soup is cooked). Finally, arrange the marigold petals and chives on top.

Narrative: Whether or not you believe in morphic resonance, the ocean of archetypal knowledge and the spiritual echo of our past lives or cellular ancestral knowledge, this dish will connect you not only to your ancestors, but to the universal wellspring of all who came before you, thereby spiritualizing your intellect and allowing you to process such deep information and understand how it is relevant to your life in the here and now.

You might serve this dish when you're pondering deep spiritual questions or want insight into the collective unconscious, so you can connect to the information encoded in your body that's been passed down by the ancestors.

🌿 Braised Kale and Cannellini Beans

1 bunch kale
2–4 tablespoons olive oil
1 or 2 pinches red pepper flakes
1 lemon, cut into wedges
4 cloves garlic, sliced thin
1 cup cooked white cannellini beans
½ cup water or broth
Salt and pepper to taste

Prepare the kale by ripping the leaves from the stalk, then breaking them into bite-size pieces. Cut the stalk into 1-inch pieces.

In a large frying pan over medium heat, warm about 2 tablespoons of olive oil, then add the kale stalks, a pinch or two of red pepper flakes, and a squeeze of lemon juice, and sauté for 3 minutes. Add the garlic, beans, and kale leaves with another squeeze of lemon juice and ½ cup water or broth. Bring to a simmer, cover, and braise until the kale is tender and the liquid has thickened, about 5 to 10 minutes. Season with salt and pepper to taste, drizzle with olive oil, and serve with the remaining lemon wedges.

Narrative: This dish offers instruction in "remembrance," passing on skills, wisdom, and ancestral knowledge, and teaching how to use this information in new ways. This is a combination of being a receptive and porous student, gleaning from family history and your own cellular memory, and finally offering the information and understanding you've collated to another person. An aspect of this is being able to clearly articulate your thoughts, being a receptive listener, and exploring concepts and ideas with others.

You might serve this dish when you start to study any new thought system in depth or are ready to share your knowledge and wisdom as a teacher.

BEING OF SERVICE

🌿 *Simple Eggplant Carpaccio*

Strictly speaking, carpaccio is an Italian hors d'oeuvre consisting of thin slices of raw beef or fish served with a sauce. Here we explore a vegetarian twist on this concept.

1 large eggplant
2 cloves garlic, finely minced
2 tablespoons extra-virgin olive oil
1–2 tablespoons freshly squeezed lemon juice
Himalayan pink salt, coarse
Freshly ground black pepper
¼ cup pine nuts, toasted
¼ cup finely chopped flat-leaf parsley
¼ cup hummus
1 ripe plum tomato, peeled and finely chopped
¼ cup plain full-fat Greek yogurt

There are several ways you can go at this. You can use the flame of a gas stove or a gas barbecue and char the eggplant over high heat. This method takes about 20 minutes and is easy. Simply char the eggplant on all sides (turning occasionally, including the top and bottom). Test for readiness by pressing the eggplant with tongs; you're feeling for a spongy softness.

The other method involves use a charcoal and woodchip barbecue. Soak a handful of hickory chips in water for 20 minutes while heating the charcoal grill. Once the grill is heated to medium-high, arrange the coals in a flat layer to create a consistent heat. Strain the hickory chips and sprinkle them over the hot coals. Wait until the smoke starts, then place the grate on the grill. Place the eggplant on the grate and, again, simply char the eggplant on all sides, turning occasionally, including the top and bottom. Test for readiness by pressing the eggplant with tongs; again, you're feeling for a spongy softness. This method is difficult to give an exact cooking time for as it depends on your grill.

Let the eggplant cool slightly. Using a knife, scrape off all the charred skin, then cut the flesh away from the seeds. The simplest way to do this is to cut off all four sides, leaving the seed core in the center. Arrange the eggplant slices one at a time on a cutting board, and using the back of a fork, flatten the eggplant until thin. Arrange the eggplant flesh (sounds very "carpaccio-ish," doesn't it?) on a platter. Then scatter the minced garlic over the eggplant, drizzle with olive oil and lemon juice, and sprinkle with salt and pepper. Finish by topping with the pine nuts and flat-leaf parsley. Serve hummus, tomato, and yogurt in small dishes on the side.

Narrative: If you've reached a place in your life where you have the time, energy, and/or finances to be of service to others but aren't sure where to start, this dish will help you explore that delightful question and find the perfect vibrational outlet for your particular gifts.

You might serve this dish when you meet with a collective of like-minded souls and want to explore together how to be of service. This vibration enhances the conversation and exploration of ideas concerning this topic, allowing all to dig deep.

EXERCISE
Intuitive Cooking

Next time you're at the market and you don't have a specific craving or a shopping list, try this intuitive cooking exercise.

1. Take a moment to settle and ask yourself, *What would I like to be nourished by?*
2. Shake out your left hand* and hover it over different foods, feeling for the strongest sensations. Allow your mind the joy of merging with each food's energy. Don't try to consciously construct a recipe as you explore.
3. Once you're ready to start cooking, take a moment to connect with the items you selected, then ask *them* how they would like to be put together, and simply follow your intuition to see what emerges.

---

*The left hand picks up information more easily than the right, as left is for receiving and right is for giving.

A wonderful aspect of this practice is looking up the food signatures of each item to find the narrative, to see what your deep self hungers for. This is a powerful way to have a conversation with your subtle body. If your intention is to cook for someone other than yourself or for a group, bring to mind those for whom you'll be cooking and simply change your question and intent to *What would most support and nourish* [name(s)]*?*

Resources

Candice Covington offers mentorships and phone sessions, or you can book an event with her.

Email: Candice@divinearchetypes.com
Website: Divine Archetypes, www.divinearchetypes.org

Hard-to-Source Eggs and Proteins
Seagull eggs: www.finefoodspecialist.co.uk
Ostrich and emu eggs: www.floeckscountry.com
Most meats and eggs listed in this book: www.fossilfarms.com

Heirloom Seeds: Unique Varieties of Common Plants
www.rareseeds.com
www.territorialseed.com

Bibliography

Baker, Ian. *The Tibetan Art of Healing.* San Francisco, Calif.: Chronicle Books, 1997.

Bolen, Jean Shinoda. *Gods in Everyman: A New Psychology of Men's Lives and Loves.* New York: HarperCollins, 1989.

Cashford, Jules. *The Moon: Myth and Image.* New York: Four Walls Eight Windows, 2002.

Chopra, Deepak. *Perfect Health: The Complete Mind/Body Guide.* New York: Three Rivers Press, 2000.

Covington, Candice. *Essential Oils in Spiritual Practice: Working with the Chakras, Divine Archetypes, and the Five Great Elements.* Rochester, Vt.: Healing Arts Press, 2017.

Frawley, Dr. David. *Ayurveda and the Mind: The Healing of Consciousness.* Twin Lakes, Wisc.: Lotus Press, 1986.

Jung, C. G. *The Archetypes and the Collective Unconscious.* Second edition. Translated by R. F. C. Hull. Bollingen Series XX. The Collected Works of C. G. Jung, volume 9, part 1. Princeton, N.J.: Princeton University Press, 1969.

Mumford, Dr. Jonn. *Magical Tattwas: A Complete System for Self-Development.* St. Paul, Minn.: Llwellyn Publications, 1997.

Porter, Valencia. *Resilient Health: How to Thrive in Our Toxic World.* Enlightened Health Media, 2018.

Sams, Jamie. *Sacred Path Cards: The Discovery of Self through Native Teachings.* New York: HarperCollins, 1990.

Tisserand, Robert B. *The Art of Aromatherapy*. Rochester, Vt.: Healing Arts Press, 1978.

Whitmont, Edward C. *The Symbolic Quest: Basic Concepts of Analytical Psychology*. New York: Putnam, 1969.

Wolkstein, Diane, and Samuel Noah Kramer. *Inanna, Queen of Heaven and Earth: Her Stories and Hymns from Sumer*. New York: Harper and Row, 1983.

Index